35
1561

Diabetes Explained:
A Layman's Guide

Diabetes Explained:
A Layman's Guide

Ira J. Laufer, M.D.
Herbert Kadison

Saturday Review Press | E. P. Dutton & Co., Inc.
New York

LIBRARY OF CONGRESS CATALOGING IN PUBLICATION DATA
Laufer, Ira J
  Diabetes explained: a layman's guide

  Bibliography: p.
  Includes index.
  1. Diabetes. I. Kadison, Herbert, joint author.
II. Title. [DNLM: 1. Diabetes mellitus. WK810 L373w]
RC660.L2 1976   616.4'62   75-38917

10 9 8 7 6 5 4 3

Published simultaneously in Canada by Clarke, Irwin & Company Limited, Toronto and Vancouver

ISBN: 0-8415-0428-8

To Irving Laufer, my father, my inspiration, my friend.

I.J.L.

To my wife, Catherine, whose forbearance and understanding
helped immeasurably.

H.K.

Contents

Diabetes Explained:
A Layman's Guide

Introduction

The material contained in this book is the natural outgrowth of a doctor-patient relationship. For a number of years the authors have functioned as doctor and patient in the diagnosis, care, and treatment of diabetes mellitus.

Over this period of time it was apparent that there were many questions that could not be answered even when the available literature was studied by a sophisticated and knowledgeable patient. The veritable explosion of knowledge in the field of diabetes made a current study of the available information almost a necessity to an understanding of this illness. In 1924 Sir Frederick Banting, the co-discoverer of insulin, stated that there is no disease that requires such intimate cooperation between the physician and patient as does diabetes mellitus. Patients, he said, should be thoroughly instructed in the cause, course, and possible complications of the disease.

His statement is even more true today, since the information now at hand, with all its ramifications, has revealed the disease to be even more intricate and more complicated than it appeared when Dr. Banting made those remarks. Diabetes is very different from most other diseases because the patient is deeply involved in his own care in a much greater way than is the doctor. For example, if an individual has pneumonia, it is really not necessary for him to know a great deal about it other than that it is an infection, that he has to take antibiotics and get a certain amount of rest, and that it will clear up after a gradual period of time. Of course, pneumonia is an acute condition and is not really the same kind of situation as diabetes, but even among chronic and long-standing diseases the patient does not really have to know much more about his condition other than that he must listen to what his physician tells him and follow the physician's dictates. In heart disease, such as angina pectoris, the patient learns that there are certain restrictions on his activities to which he must subscribe, and that there are certain medications he must take. There are dietary regulations, perhaps, and certain restraints on his emotional ability and on his way of life, but the path he must tread is considerably much less narrow than that followed by the patient with diabetes.

The diabetic patient is living with a severe metabolic abnormality twenty-four hours a day, seven days a week, and he has to learn early on of the many influences that can have an effect on what may be essentially a precarious balance, depending on the severity of the case and the individual concerned. Emotional upset, dietary irregularities, exercise, other medications, the use of insulin, with certain of its complications, are some of the factors that may change rapidly from moment to moment. And each has separate and distinct reactions in the patient. The diabetic must be aware of these and how they affect him in order to keep himself in as good a metabolic equilibrium as possible so that he will be able to live a fruitful and useful life and perhaps avert the onset of the complications of diabetes.

1

The Enemy

If you are under the illusion that diabetes is not a deadly enemy of mankind, rampant in the world and increasing in its magnitude each year, ponder this incontrovertible fact—diabetes is now the fifth leading cause of disease-related death in the United States when only at the turn of the century it ranked twenty-seventh on that grim list. While you are giving some serious thought to that reality, you might also consider that there are about five million people in the United States today who do not even know that they are diabetic.

And perhaps, if the number of deaths from heart disease, arteriosclerotic disease, kidney failure, and cerebrovascular accidents (strokes) were traced back to their root causes, it would be found that many were due to complications or effects of long-term diabetes, diagnosed or undiagnosed, on the

3

cardiovascular system and the kidneys. In its annual summary for 1973 the Bureau of Vital Statistics of the United States Public Health Service listed 359 deaths per 100,000 population as attributable to heart disease, 102 deaths per 100,000 to strokes, and 17 per 100,000 resulting from diabetes. It also reported that there were 35,000 deaths listing diabetes as the single cause. Were each of the deaths listed as caused by heart disease or stroke to be investigated thoroughly, it might well be found that diabetes was a contributing factor of major proportion, and this would probably move the disease to an even higher position on the list of causes of death.

A classic example was the death of famed baseball star Jackie Robinson, in 1972, from a heart attack. However, Mr. Robinson had suffered for some twenty years from diabetes and had developed most of the conditions that can arise after long-term affliction with the disease. He had lost the sight of one eye and was becoming progressively blind in the other. Pains in his legs from diabetic damage to the arteries and nerves had caused him to give up his favorite recreation, golf, because he found it too uncomfortable to walk long distances. All in all, the combination of factors resulting from the progressive damage done by diabetes finally brought on the fatal heart attack that was listed as Mr. Robinson's cause of death. Given knowledge of his medical history, though, many physicians would list his death as occurring from complications of diabetes, thus adding it to the growing list of such fatalities.

In support of this are the results of a study conducted by the Pennsylvania Health Department indicating that some 300,000 diabetics die each year in the United States, not the 35,000 whose cause of death is officially listed as diabetes. In fact, the conclusions were that diabetes could be considered the third leading cause rather than the fifth if deaths in which it was present but unreported were added to those where it was listed as the underlying or contributing cause.

Dr. George K. Tokuhata reported these conclusions to the 1974 meeting of the American Public Health Association.

Dr. Tokuhata, director of the Pennsylvania Health Department's Bureau of Program Evaluation, and professor of epidemiology and biostatistics at the University of Pittsburgh Graduate School of Public Health, reported that:

A. Of some 200,000 death certificates reviewed, 10,170 mentioned diabetes as a cause of death; 2,639 recorded it as the underlying cause, 7,531 as a contributory cause.

B. When a random sample of the certifying physicians who had not listed diabetes on the death certificate were asked specifically to list all diseases and conditions diagnosed in their patients, it was found that 8 in 100 patients whose cause of death did not include diabetes on their death certificates did, in fact, have diabetes.

Applying this rate of hidden or unreported cases of diabetes to the total number of deaths resulting from all other causes, Dr. Tokuhata estimated that there were 8,800 additional Pennsylvanians who had diabetes at the time of death. He further noted that if these statistics were applied to the entire United States, nearly 304,000 people would be expected to die annually with diabetes rather than the now-accepted 35,000.

In further corroboration, the report of the National Commission on Diabetes published in December, 1975, stated that when diabetes and its complications are considered together, it emerges as the third leading cause of death in the United States. "Mortality statistics do not generally specify underlying or contributing cause of death, resulting in a lack of accurate information on the actual death rate from diabetes," said the report.

While the Robinson case may be a textbook example, physicians recognize that diabetes is a most mysterious disease and may not uniformly act as anticipated. It may attack without warning with the standard symptoms of fatigue, excessive thirst, frequent urination, rapid loss of weight, high blood sugar content, itching, and, sometimes, sexual impotence in males. It may also lie completely dormant, exhibiting no symptoms whatsoever until precipitated by one of the many factors that can trigger its onset.

The extreme opposite of the Robinson case existed in an uncle of one of the authors. Uncle Jack was diagnosed as diabetic at the age of fifty-five and simply refused to accept the condition as a good reason to change his activities, diet, or life-style. He continued to eat as he pleased, and to take his medication when and if he thought of it, and practically ignored his chronic illness. To everyone's amazement, he lived until the age of eighty-four and enjoyed every moment of his ostensibly carefree life!

Citing two such extreme examples—and they are by no means unusual—it is no wonder that medical researchers and practitioners say that diabetes is an enemy not easily understood, whose variations in onset and manifestations have not yet been fathomed. The disease now exists in "have-not" cultures as well as in affluent societies, when it was originally thought to be the result of high living and overindulgence in both food and drink. Diabetes has been recognized as a disease entity since the earliest times of recorded history, and still comparatively little is known about its mode of action.

For years scientists have been grappling with questions which, for the most part, still disclose no definitive answers:

- ·· Why does arteriosclerotic disease occur much earlier in diabetics than in the normal population?
- ·· What is the inheritance pattern for the diabetic tendency?
- ·· What is the basic defect inherited by the person destined to become diabetic?
- ·· What is the relative importance of heredity versus environmental factors?
- ·· What is the best criterion of metabolic defect, particularly in the earlier stages of the diabetic state?

·· Is there some other marker to be found early on in the disease process that precedes and is more reliable than mild abnormalities of sugar utilization in predicting the future development of diabetes in a particular individual?

·· Why is it that the complications that beset Jackie Robinson do not appear in some other diabetics, thus permitting them to live out a reasonably normal life-span in comparative comfort?

·· With diabetes now the third leading cause of new blindness in the United States, because of damage to the retina of the eye and cataracts, why is it that many diabetics do not suffer this condition?

·· Is there something unique about diabetes that causes it to affect the smallest arteries?

·· What is the mechanism in diabetes that results in a decreased ability to handle bacterial infections?

·· Why do the cells of diabetics age faster than those of normal people?

Perhaps when the answers to these and other questions posed by the disease are answered, this new information will shed light on some of the other medical problems facing mankind. Some researchers are of the opinion that when more is known about diabetes, it will increase the knowledge of the aging process in man.

According to the National Health Interview Survey of 1965–66, the last comprehensive determination of the number of diabetics in the United States, it was estimated that about 4.4 million persons in this country have diabetes. By applying statistical analysis to the raw data it was also estimated that about 1.6 million of these do not even know they have the disease, and probably had not yet developed symptoms, and that some might not have been sufficiently aware of the symptoms manifested for them to seek medical care.

The survey disclosed that unsuspected diabetes is found with greater frequency among older persons, the obese, and relatives of diabetics, and it is ten times more frequent after age forty-five. About 320,000 persons each year learn for the first time that they have the disease. It is most prevalent among low-income groups, with the rate of incidence in families with under $4,000 annual income being more than double that in families with higher incomes. And it is most prevalent in nonwhite females over the age of forty-five. According to testimony given in 1973 before the U.S. Senate Subcommittee on Health, the incidence of diabetes has doubled during the last decade.

After the National Health Interview Survey had compiled its statistics, it was conservatively estimated that the annual cost of the disease in the United States alone was $2 billion. This includes the time lost by diabetics from gainful employment as well as the actual medical and hospital expenses for treatment. By applying a reasonable rate of inflation to the costs as given in 1966, one might easily arrive at a current annual cost of about $4 billion.

Epidemiologists and statisticians, working with figures provided by various health organizations, estimate that by now diabetes afflicts at least 5 percent of the world's population.

Why is diabetes on the increase? Historically it seemed to be a disease that followed affluence and was related to food intake. It was noted by Willis in the 1600s that its appearance or manifestation occurred after increased ingestion of rich food and wines. Physicians during the Siege of Paris in the late 1800s, when food was scarce and diet restricted, noted that the number of cases of diabetes decreased, and this was also found to be true during World War II, when food was rationed and diet was limited in both amount and variety. Most adults with diabetes are overweight, and they improve by losing avoirdupois. And as society has become more affluent, as more civilizations have moved from "have-not" to "have" status, more diabetes is becoming apparent. Then, how to relate this to the statistic that people in the lowest economic bracket show the most diabetes? It may well be that this group subsists mainly on a diet high in carbohydrates, the metabolism of which is a prime factor in diabetes, because that kind of food is cheaper and more readily available than the protein foods. This results in their being fat but malnourished, a condition that has been described as "potato fat."

Diabetes also tends to be related to stress and to urbanization. People have been living for many years in a time of increased world stress, with the threat of nuclear holocaust ever somewhere in the back of the mind, when life itself has become so complicated that many people find it difficult to cope. As concerns life-style and its influence on diabetes, the rate of the disease in Rhodesia, Africa, was very low until more and more of the people during the past two decades moved from the bush to the cities. Their diets changed, the stresses of their daily living increased, their physical activity decreased, and today diabetes is more common among this population. They are victims of civilization, of eating more and better refined foods, and of a more sedentary existence. According to a study by A. C. B. Wicks, W. M. Castle, and M. Gelfand of the University of Rhodesia in Salisbury, the particular villain in the diet was the greater amount of refined carbohydrates in the city diet as opposed to the normal bush diet, in which the carbohydrate, although high, was of the type that was less refined and that became absorbed in the bloodstream more slowly.

Although clinical diabetes is still rare among Eskimos, more of them showed some of the disease's symptomatology in 1972 than was true ten years earlier. This was an increase in difficulty of carbohydrate metabolism that does not appear to have a genetic basis but may instead be associated with physical activity and physical fitness. In the last ten years Eskimos have made increasing use of labor-saving devices—snow machines instead of dog sleds, chain saws instead of hand saws, and fuel oil instead of wood for heat. These factors may have decreased their physical activity and fitness. Physical fitness is associated with less obesity and an increased muscle mass. The latter may result in faster tissue utilization of glucose and an enhanced metabolism of this substance.

Dr. G. D. Campbell of the King Edward VIII Hospital in Durban, Natal, South Africa, reported at the International Diabetes Federation meeting in 1970 that where quantity and particularly the quality of food changes, as in a previously rural people now living in civilized areas, then there appears an additional rate of diabetes that is often very high indeed.

In the East Indians and Bantus in South Africa there is a trend toward large intake of refined carbohydrate foods when they live in the cities. It appeared to Campbell that the increased incidence of diabetes in this population is due to the quality of carbohydrate, which he considers as a determinant of the emergence of diabetes. The people of the lower class were obese with a diet very high in refined carbohydrate —over 75 percent. And, relating diet to activity, the East Indians habitually conserved energy by moving slowly with never an unnecessary movement. Thus energy expenditure and caloric utilization were very low.

People who live on home-pounded cereals (which are unrefined carbohydrate mainly) suffer only what Dr. Campbell describes as "background" or "essential" frequency of diabetes. He remarked that it is most noticeable how the positions of the highest frequency of diabetes in the statistics have recently been filled by dark-skinned people. In many instances, such as in East Indians all over the world, those remaining at home with their traditional and familiar diet have a much smaller comparative frequency of diabetes, linked to a lower rate of obesity.

American Indian tribes in the Southwest United States have shown an increasing rate of diabetes among adults over the past thirty-five years.

Dr. Kelly M. West of the University of Oklahoma College

of Medicine stated in the journal *Diabetes* in late 1974 that among Indian tribes in Oklahoma roughly one third of the full-blooded tribe members over age thirty have diabetes.

He found that the common features revealed by his study were:

1. Diabetes was probably rare in all tribes prior to 1940.
2. Diabetes is now common in all.
3. All tribes were previously slender.
4. All are now fat.

Many researchers in medicine, epidemiologists, and bio-statisticians have reviewed the health status of American Indian tribes and almost uniformly report that diabetes was a rarity until the 1940s. Extensive review of medical reports by the civilian and military physicians serving the Oklahoma Indians between 1832 and 1939 revealed no evidence of the presence of diabetes. According to Dr. West, in contrast to the situation in many native populations the Oklahoma tribes had, for the most part, considerable medical attention in the nineteenth and early twentieth centuries, often by the same physicians who were finding diabetes common in their white patients.

A report of the Division of Indian Health in 1963 showed that the diabetes-related death rate in white persons in the United States between forty-five and fifty-four years of age was 12.1 per 100,000 while in Indians the rate was 59.3. Dr. West comments that a substantial portion of the increase is doubtless attributable to better screening and diagnostic programs, but there is considerable evidence to suggest that much of this increase is real. In 1955 there was no significant difference between Indians and whites in diabetes-related deaths. By 1967 the rate among Indians was 2.3 times that among the white population.

To reemphasize the mysterious manner in which diabetes

acts, there is considerable difference in prevalence of the disease among the Indian tribes. In 1966 Maurice L. Seivers, chief of the department of medicine, Public Health Service Indian Hospital, Phoenix, Arizona, reported that among adult Indians admitted to the medical service of the hospital 45 percent of the Pimas and 33 percent of the Colorado River and 32 percent of the Papago tribe had diabetes. These contrast with 9.7 percent and 1 percent with diabetes among the Hopi and Navajo admissions. While hospital admissions cannot be assumed to reflect true prevalence rates, such marked differences must reflect either variations in true prevalence or major differences in morbidity from diabetes among these tribes, or a combination of both factors.

Dr. West further noted that the Oklahoma tribes, particularly, are of interest because of the great diversity of their geographic, cultural, and genetic origins. These tribes originated from all parts of the continent. Some of the Oklahoma tribes are related to tribes from other areas in which rates of diabetes are high, and some are related to those in which diabetes is uncommon. Before their removal to Oklahoma in the nineteenth century, some had been nomadic hunters and meat eaters who had been on low-carbohydrate diets for centuries, while others had derived a substantial portion of their daily food from starches. Interestingly, in photographs taken of Oklahoma Indians in the latter part of the nineteenth century one can see that they were very lean. Now the middle-aged men tend to be fat and the middle-aged women very fat.

In other cultures diabetes appears to be on the increase. The history of the disease in the Polynesian people is strikingly similar in several respects to that in the American Indians and Eskimos. Increasing rates were first observed in the Maoris of New Zealand and native Hawaiians. It seems to be concurrent with the degree of adiposity. It also seems to relate to the amount of acculturation present in change of diet and adaptation of life-style from the manner in which they lived as primitive people to reflect more closely the Western-type civilization. There is some uncertainty about the origin of Polynesians, Micronesians, and Melanesians, but most experts have concluded that they migrated west to east from lands in or nearer Asia than their present domiciles. Thus they appear to share with Eskimos and American Indians an Asian origin and so a common genetic background.

Dr. G. Mimura of the Kumamoto University in Japan reported to the International Diabetes Federation in 1970 that the general incidence of diabetes in Japan is slightly lower than in European-American countries. Recently the food supply has increased, owing to betterment of the economic situation, and with this increase has come a rise in the rate of diabetes. The same pattern was noted by Dr. L. Travia of the National Institute for Diabetes and Metabolic Disease in Rome, Italy, who correlated deaths from diabetes with economic conditions and the availability of consumption goods. His statistics indicate a drop in the death rate when the economy in Italy worsened. He also stated, however, that the incidence of diabetes in the world has increased in the last seventy-five years. In 1900, he says, there were 1,082 deaths, or 3.3 per 100,000, while in 1965 there were 9,396 deaths, or 17.8 per 100,000. Another Italian medical researcher indicated a correlation between the mortality rate and the total caloric value of the diet. In 1900, in Italy, the total calories consumed per day averaged 2,500, and in 1965 the caloric intake averaged 2,840. Although there was only a 17 percent increase in total calories, there was a 500 percent increase in mortality. Thus perhaps diet played a part but not the whole role. Inquiries concerning the diet of diabetics before the onset of disease revealed that for several years prior to onset these patients' diets had been excessive, beyond the theoretical requirements based on the expenditure of energy caused by physical and occupational activities.

Dr. Jean Mayer of Harvard University, the noted expert on

nutrition, wrote in his syndicated column in June, 1975, that a group of researchers in Israel in 1961 had studied the prevalence of diabetes among two ethnic groups living in Israel. Among Sephardic Jews (of Spanish origin) the rate was 1 percent, while among the Ashkenazi (of Eastern European extraction) it was 2½ percent.

Among 5,000 new immigrants to Israel there were only 3 cases, but among Yemenite Jews who had lived in Israel twenty-five years or more the incidence was higher than among the Ashkenazi. Similar findings were observed when new immigrant Kurdish Jews were compared to Kurdish old settlers. A dietary survey revealed that in Yemen the people consumed almost no table sugar, whereas in Israel a considerable percentage of the carbohydrate intake was in the form of sugar. The same kind of dietary change was noted in the Kurdish Jews.

While environmental and social factors have played an important role in the increase, there is a genetic tendency that appears to govern its passage from generation to generation. How this works, just where the genetic fault lies, and what bodily process it influences are still unknown, but the tendency does exist. It is known that relatives of diabetics are three times more apt to contract the disease than people in whose families it has not appeared.

While obesity has been linked to diabetes (85 percent of all diabetics are overweight), not all fat people become diabetic. Pregnancy or certain infections may precipitate the disease in some individuals, but not all pregnant women or people who suffer infections become diabetics. No, there appears to be another factor which, because it is known that diabetes runs in families, must be related to heredity.

As in many genetically influenced diseases, some who possess the tendency will themselves become overt diabetics and others will merely pass the susceptibility on to their offspring without manifesting the disease themselves.

In describing the hereditary aspects of diabetes, according to Mendelian laws on inheritance, the following expectancies are accepted by the geneticists:

1. A carrier is an individual, male or female, who, although free of a disease, transmits to his or her offspring the tendency to, or the potentiality for, the disease from his or her ancestors.

2. When a diabetic marries a nondiabetic who is not a carrier, it is almost certain that none of their children will develop diabetes, but they will be carriers.

3. In a marriage of two carriers, 25 percent of their children will be diabetic; 75 percent will be carriers.

4. When a diabetic marries a carrier, 50 percent of their children will become diabetic, and 50 percent will be carriers.

5. If two diabetics marry, all of their children will become diabetic eventually.

This rather oversimplified genetic description does not hold in all cases. There are many other factors in the patient's environment and behavior which change the emergence of the disease.

It is estimated that one quarter of the population—some 50 million people—in the United States are carriers. According to the National Center for Health Statistics, while diabetes is found in families it may skip a generation or more in its appearance. Diabetes occurred in three successive generations in only one percent of the diabetic population. One out of six had diabetic mothers, and one out of twelve had diabetic fathers. One out of four of those with brothers or sisters knew of at least one brother or sister who also had diabetes.

Look for a moment at some other reasons why diabetes appears to be on the increase.

First, there is a general increase in life expectancy because of new knowledge in disease prevention, public health procedures that stave off fatal epidemics, and more sophisticated medical knowledge generally. Thus people all over the world are living longer, and it is known that diabetes tends to appear with aging. The discovery of insulin and its widespread use among juvenile-onset diabetics increased their life-span so that they reached childbearing age and transmitted the diabetic tendency to their descendants. If, twenty or thirty years ago, someone had pneumonia and died at the age of thirty because of the lack of antibiotic medication, he may not have manifested diabetes but may have had the genetic tendency, which he transmitted to his offspring.

Second, case finding is better today than it was in the past, from the standpoint of both the patient and the physician. The patient is influenced because there is greater emphasis now on good health, on preventive medicine, on undergoing regular examinations. Patients are submitting themselves to good medical diagnosis at a time when physicians are utilizing increasingly sophisticated means to determine diabetes. Years ago the diagnosis would be established merely by testing the urine for sugar—a very gross test because diabetes can be present with a negative urine sugar but a high blood sugar content. Today physicians' tests are better and blood sugar content is being determined in various ways, with even more elaborate procedures available now than previously.

Third, people who suspect they may have diabetes are going to physicians more readily now because they know that oral medication is available and is effective in certain cases. In the past the fear of finding out that they had diabetes, which would then have to be treated by injected insulin, kept many people from going to a physician to have their suspicions about the disease confirmed. The oral hypoglycemic drugs tended to reduce the fear of finding out, so case identification became enhanced.

There is also an increase in the rate of complications resulting from long-term diabetes because insulin and other measures have enabled the diabetic to live long enough to show the sequelae. Fifty years ago the diabetic did not survive to suffer some of the things that develop ten, twenty, and thirty years after onset of the disease. So the apparent increase in complications may be merely due to the fact the improved overall treatment enables diabetics to live a nearly normal life-span. The advent of the antibiotic drugs has enabled potential diabetics to overcome what used to be fatal diseases and thus to live long enough to develop diabetes.

The present and future dangers of the disease as well as its rising prevalence in the world have resulted in its now being studied most intensively among all of the endocrine diseases, not only with improved treatment as the immediate goal but with the long-term aim of finding the basic cause in order to prevent its occurrence. The mystery of diabetes extends not only to its pathology and physiology but also to its course and manifestations. It is one condition that requires the total commitment of the patient to his treatment and total cooperation with his physician if he wants to improve. As in dealing with many complicated matters, first things are first, and so it is in diabetes. The early needs are to control the sugar content of the blood, to stop urinating so much, to clear the vision, to feel stronger, and to normalize the weight. Once these immediate problems are alleviated and the patient is in balance, the next concern is with the long-term degenerative effects of the disease on the vascular system, the eyes, the kidneys, and the nervous system.

While the beneficial effects of good control on the ultimate complications are still being debated vigorously in the medical community, there is increasing evidence that the maintenance of a proper balance of blood sugar does have a mitigating effect on the complications of diabetes.

A recent report from the famed Joslin Clinic in Boston, in which a study of forty-year survivors of diabetes was undertaken, challenges the inevitability of the degenerative changes—blindness, leg gangrene, heart disorders, kidney failure. The report concluded that if carbohydrate balance is well maintained, most diabetics suffer only minor complications.

Dr. H. T. Hsu of the Joslin Clinic reported on a study of 73 juvenile-onset diabetics who were followed from the time of diagnosis, which was prior to the age of fifteen in each case. They had all lived with the disease at least forty years. Well over half of them had had at least one episode of ketoacidosis, the most accentuated form of blood sugar elevation accompanied by other biochemical imbalances in the body. By accepted standards in diabetology many should have been severely disabled, but their medical records and the medical examination given in 1966 and 1967 revealed this not to be so. A noteworthy characteristic of the study group, Dr. Hsu believes, is the relatively low rate of vascular problems, considering the length of the illness. This is important, he said, in view of the unanimous agreement among other published studies that damage to the arterial blood vessels increases in proportion to length of illness. Whether maintenance of rigid glucose balance actually lowers the incidence of blood vessel problems among juvenile-onset diabetics remains controversial, and the Joslin researchers are not claiming that good control was the sole source of success with the group studied. But they do feel that "conscientious regulation played a major role in these patients' long-term survival with relatively minor complications."

Another Joslin researcher, Dr. Alexander Marble, in reporting to the International Diabetes Federation meeting in 1970, said:

> I believe that there is good evidence to suggest that the vascular disease of diabetes is secondary to a metabolic defect, namely insulin deficiency. This point of view

transforms the outlook for the diabetic from one of de-spair to one of hope. This makes the early detection and treatment of diabetes logical rather than a pointless waste of time. If one accepts this orientation, then it is the re-sponsibility of the physician to treat each patient as care-fully and as well as the individual situation may allow. This implies treatment not only to the extent of abolishing characteristic symptoms but also of maintaining as good "chemical control" as practicable. In this way, I believe that the vascular complications of long-term diabetes may at least be postponed or minimized.

Diabetes is vastly different from other diseases because the patient is deeply involved in his own care to an extent that does not exist in almost any other chronic illness. The condi-tion can extend over a lifetime, and there is no other ailment that so intimately involves the total metabolism as does dia-betes. In other endocrine disorders where there is necessity to replace hormones—pituitary insufficiency, lack of thyroid, or adrenal aberration—the patient takes his prescribed replace-ment medication and worries about little else. The diabetic, on the other hand, is affected for good or ill by many influ-ences—dietary matters, emotional disturbances, infections, the necessity for medications that may affect blood sugar content, to name but a few. While other diseases are chronic, they are not as chronic as diabetes. And the patient's behav-ior at various stages may have an effect on what happens to him ten or twenty years later.

The patient is forced to be deeply involved in his own care in order to understand the things that can upset his balance, because what the physician attempts to do in diabetic man-agement is to maintain the blood sugar level within relatively restricted ranges, as the nondiabetic does naturally. The phy-sician prescribes for the patient methods by which this can be accomplished—dietary regime, medication, exercise, and a calm, well-ordered way of life. The balance is really very difficult because of the many factors that can cause the diabetic to break out of the restricted way of life that keeps the blood sugar within acceptable limits.

Many times, diabetes will manifest itself after extreme emotional stress or crisis, or it can be intensified by the same causes. Dietary indiscretion is an obvious reason for imbalance—straying from the prescribed food or drink will pour more sugar into the body, and stability then goes out the window. Physical exercise is a big factor in controlling the blood sugar level because increased muscular activity lowers blood sugar. The balance may be disturbed by an infection such as pneumonia or incipient appendicitis brewing in the body. Medications prescribed for high blood pressure or for arthritis may also increase the blood sugar.

In addition to those factors, there are others to think about. What happens in traveling long distances by airplane with the resultant "jet lag" and disturbance to body rhythms? What does one do when visiting other countries where the food is vastly different from the regular diet? The vital and fundamental thing that the diabetic must always keep in mind is that his abnormality is constantly with him, is related to and changes in relationship to everything he is doing. Not all diabetics need to consider all of these factors all of the time, but all must bear them in mind some of the time. The diabetic must always be mindful that, even if his balance is good, the stimuli that can tip the scales one way or another, sometimes with disastrous results, are many and varied.

However, even though the world faces a dangerous and complex enemy in diabetes, it is on the threshold of a whole new era in understanding the nature of the disease and in control of its long-term complications. During the forty years following the discovery and utilization of insulin there had really not been a great deal of new knowledge unearthed because the widespread use of insulin had conveyed the belief that the cure was here. However, a method for measuring circulating insulin in the blood was perfected in 1950, and it was found that some diabetics did produce insulin, so it seemed that the diabetic fault lay somewhere else in the process of insulin's action. This has led to a whole new approach to the study of diabetes, ranging from the source of the insulin in the pancreas to the effect of insulin at the cell level.

The primary aim of diabetic management is to try to do in the diabetic what the normal individual does naturally— maintaining the blood sugar level within narrow and acceptable bounds at all times. Even with the best of contemporary treatment this is not always possible; other means of maintaining the proper insulin-sugar ratio are therefore being studied at an accelerated rate. In addition, studies of the basic causes of diabetes are going on at a frenetic pace.

And well they might.

The sooner some real progress is made toward finding out why diabetes occurs the better. At its present rate of proliferation, it is possible that some time in the future diabetes will afflict everyone in the world.

At the very best the condition is debilitating; at the worst it is the cause of considerable suffering and untimely death. In some cases, notably in children, its ferocity knows no bounds, while in others it can be relatively benign. However, ferocious or tame, those with the disease are affected over their entire lifetime. They must modify their life-styles to accommodate the disease.

The cost in real monetary terms is now great. Further increased incidence could make the cost enormous, even overwhelming, to the economy. Its effect on the health care resources also could be such as to strain them beyond their capacity to provide ameliorative measures. To say that diabetes is one of the most pressing public health problems in the world today would not overstate the case.

There is no doubt but that the face of this dangerous enemy of mankind takes on many disguises and appears to be a mystery that is as yet unsolvable. But medicine is ever hopeful and ever anxious to unravel the most complicated of problems—and diabetes certainly falls into that category.

2

The History

Diabetes mellitus as an enemy of mankind is of ancient origin. It was first described in the Ebers Papyrus, dated about 1500 B.C., wherein a medical prescription is described for the relief of polyuria, frequent urination. This is considered to be the first allusion to diabetes mellitus in the recorded history of medicine. A few centuries later, other papyri also contained recipes to relieve polyuria. It can only be inferred that the disease must have antedated these written records by some undetermined time. Even the sketchy information that has survived through the years indicates that it was noticed very early by ancient Egyptian and Greek physicians. Their limited knowledge but boundless imagination, combined with powers of observation and some insight, brought them to conclusions and data that are as valid now as they were hundreds, even thousands, of years ago.

Since it is now known that the high blood sugar content typical in diabetes causes excessive urination along with other effects, it might be interesting to speculate for a moment about the disease's original development in man and how it appeared in the genetic code of the first sufferer, who then passed it on to his or her descendants. This is, of course, granting that the tendency to diabetes is inherited according to the accepted laws of heredity. In nature, aberrations of this sort are usually a response to a specific stimulus or need for the particular characteristic, which will then overcome or mitigate a damaging condition. For example, the sickling of the red blood cells in some blacks was found to protect against the common malaria in Africa. Now that this protective device is no longer needed in the black population living in the United States, its presence is cause for concern among those who may still carry the sickle-cell anemia trait.

As far as the origin of diabetes is concerned, in very ancient times when food was hard to come by and a high blood sugar was necessary to provide the energy to cope with the day-to-day struggle for existence, perhaps those who carried above-normal blood sugars survived better. Perhaps they were stronger and more capable of surviving the rigors of life. Perhaps this led to the creation of a gene for high blood sugar, thus beginning the descent of diabetes through the generations to the present day. There is no way, of course, to prove this theory, but it is something to consider when attempting to determine what diabetes is doing here.

The first clinical description of the disease was given in the second century A.D. by a Greek physician, Aretaeus of Cappadocia. He named the condition ''diabetes'' when he observed that a great amount of urine was passed. The word *diabetes* in Ionic Greek meant ''a siphon.''

Aretaeus wrote:

> Diabetes is a wonderful afflication, not very frequent among men, being a melting down of the flesh and limbs

into urine. The patients never stop making water, but the flow is incessant as if opening an aqueduct. Life is short, disgusting and painful; thirst unquenchable, excessive drinking which, however, is disproportionate to the large quantity of urine, for more urine is passed; and one cannot stop them either from drinking or making water. Or if for a time they abstain from drinking, their mouth becomes parched and their body dry; the viscera seems as if scorched up; they are affected with nausea, restlessness and burning thirst; and at no distant term they expire.

He also speaks of primary and secondary appearance of the malady:

The cause of it may be that someone who has the disease may have left some malignity lurking in the past. It is not improbable, also, that something pernicious, derived from other diseases which attack the bladder and kidneys may sometimes prove the cause of this afflication.

This ancient scholar was not far off the track in this observation since it is now known that diabetes mellitus often makes its first appearance not only after injury or mental shock but also after a bout of acute disease such as influenza or pneumonia. In children, especially, it may occur after any of the infectious diseases common in childhood. The ancient physicians had no body of real scientific knowledge on which to rely because chemistry was virtually unknown and biochemistry not even dreamed of. However, almost to a man they correctly noted the symptoms and observed that the diabetic's urine was sweet and attracted flies.

Some, especially those in India, described signs that are recognized today as those of ketosis, which is the acute accentuation of the symptoms of diabetes with blood sugars much higher than usual for a particular patient. In this condition there is a production of what are called ketone bodies, which result in profound changes in the body chemistry, often leading to death. The Indian physicians also noted the onset of diabetic coma preceding death. They were quick to correlate diabetes with overweight and considered it a disease of rich and greedy persons whose diet was high in rice, starchy food, and sugar. They did not project their thinking to recommend treating diabetes by controlling the diet. Had they done so, perhaps this might have pointed the way for others to prescribe nutrition habits that would have aided the diabetics of that era.

Paracelsus, a European who lived from 1493 to 1541, evaporated the urine of a diabetic and found a residue of white powder. It is unfortunate that he mistook this for salt and concluded that it was the salt that caused a great amount of urination. Had he identified it correctly as sugar, the study of diabetes might well have taken a giant step forward.

Because little was known about body metabolism, the relationship of carbohydrate intake to the production of sugar was never, up to that time, studied scientifically. However, Thomas Sydenham, called the "English Hippocrates," who lived between 1624 and 1689, noted that diabetics did very well on a meat diet (high in protein) and that their urine sugar often disappeared.

As chemistry advanced, it was possible in 1766 for Matthew Dobson to observe definitely that the sweetness of urine was due to the presence of sugar. Many of the known manifestations of the disease were then observed and recorded: tendency toward boils and carbuncles, ulcerations of the feet and lower limbs, gangrene, diabetic coma, air hunger as part of the diabetic coma, retinitis (degeneration in the retina of the eye), and acidosis (abnormal acidity in the body).

During the scientific surge of the late nineteenth century, scientists all over the world were pursuing many paths of research into medical problems, and diabetes was being studied intensely because of the mystery surrounding both its inception and course. Paul Langerhans in 1869 first noted cells in clusters throughout the pancreas that were different in formation and appearance from the other pancreatic cells. These have become known as the islets of Langerhans, but at that time their insulin-secreting property was not discerned.

The year 1889 marked a milestone in discovery when two medical scientists, J. Von Mering and Oscar Minkowski, became interested in finding out what would happen after a dog's pancreas was removed. And here enters one of those accidents, serendipity if you will, in which researchers obtain a result far from the original aim. In this particular experiment Von Mering and Minkowski were studying the digestion of fats and were curious concerning the effect the absence of the pancreas would have on that process. They carried out their experiments on a number of dogs and found that they all developed the classic symptoms of diabetes mellitus. This located the site of the cause of diabetes indubitably in the pancreas.

Although the pancreas had been known since the days of the early Greek physicians, understanding of its function was not complete. Many medical scholars ascribed different reasons for its presence in the body, most of which were not correct.

It should be noted that in 1683 a Swiss named Johann Conrad Brunner removed the pancreas from dogs and kept them alive. He noted great thirst and excessive urination but did not identify this as diabetes mellitus. His work was the first involving the internal secretions of the pancreas, but his observations went mostly unnoticed or disregarded.

In 1893 E. G. Laguesse and E. Hedon suspected, in following up the work of Langerhans, that the islets constituted the endocrine portion of the pancreas, providing the internal secretion of that organ.

One work led to another, and in 1899 Diamare found that there were two types of cells in the islets. In 1902 Eugene L. Opie, while working in the pathological-anatomical laboratory at Johns Hopkins University in Baltimore, performed autopsies on diabetics and found pronounced degeneration of the islets of Langerhans. The same observation was made independently by other scientists. It was later proved that even atrophy of the pancreas did not affect the islets, nor did diabetes occur. If, however, the islets were injured, diabetic symptoms appeared immediately. Thus, building on the results provided by Von Mering and Minkowski that loss of the entire pancreas resulted in the appearance of diabetes, the direction taken by research was toward isolating beyond a doubt the area in the pancreas important in diabetes.

In 1907 M. A. Lane described the two types of islet cells as Type A and Type B and de Mayer in 1909 named the B cell secretion insulin. In 1915 J. Homan confirmed that the Type B cells secrete insulin, but this was considered as still hypothetical at that time. Sir Edward Sharpey-Schafer began, in 1916, to believe that the islets produced a substance that controlled the metabolism of carbohydrates. He, too, suggested the name insulin for this hypothetical hormone.

The most important accomplishment in diabetes management, the isolation of a pure extract of insulin and its application to a human diabetic, took place on July 30, 1921, the work of Dr. Frederick G. Banting and medical student Charles H. Best, in Toronto, Canada. What they did turned the problem of diabetes around 180 degrees. It promised a reasonably normal existence and improved life-span for diabetics who were previously doomed to an early death while living literally a hell on earth. The notes of Banting and Best state that they gave the hormone the name Isletin, but Professor J. J. R. Macleod, in whose laboratory they performed their experiments, insisted that it should be called insulin, and so it remains.

Banting, a native Canadian, originally thought he would be a minister but turned to medicine when he decided that a career in the cloth was not to his liking. He became a military surgeon during World War I, and his duties enabled him to polish his surgical technique. After the war he began practicing orthopedic surgery, but his practice was not as busy as it might have been, so he spent his spare time reading medical literature. He became interested in the problem of diabetes after studying the work of Von Mering and Minkowski, theorizing that if the pancreas were the controlling factor in the disease it must be possible somehow to isolate the substance that maintained normal metabolism.

He discussed his ideas with Dr. J. J. R. Macleod of the University of Toronto, whom he persuaded to provide laboratory space and experimental animals. Dr. Macleod also recruited Charles H. Best, a senior student in physiology and biochemistry, to be Dr. Banting's assistant. Best was born in Maine, although his parents were Canadian, and his father was a physician. Best early on showed an interest in medicine and entered Toronto University as a medical student after service during World War I.

Tribute must be paid to those scientists through the years whose inquisitive minds and fertile imaginations paved the way for Banting and Best to conduct their experiments and to meet with success. What Banting added to the work that preceded his was the theory that an extract of the pancreas's external secretion destroyed the secretion of the islet cells when taken together. Banting and Best then blocked the pancreatic ducts in an innovative fashion, causing complete degeneration of the organ section that excreted the external digestive secretion. They were then able to take a pure secretion from the islets of Langerhans.

With the insulin thus obtained, Banting and Best succeeded in lowering the blood sugar of a diabetic for the first time in history. The first patient to receive insulin was an eleven-year-old diabetic named Leonard Thompson, whose disease had been diagnosed two years previously. On a 450-calorie-a-day diet, he was down to 75 pounds. After insulin injection he improved markedly, living to maturity.

Banting and Best then injected insulin into a physician

named Joseph Gilchrist, who only a short time previously had exhibited the symptoms of diabetes. He willingly subjected himself to the experiments with the newly isolated substance. Every new specimen of insulin was tried on him, to the point where he sometimes suffered from excessive doses and resultant insulin shock, with hypoglycemia, mental confusion, and weakness. As a physician, he was able to give Banting and Best a complete description of that condition, the first account of it in medical history.

While Banting and Best were hailed as the discoverers of insulin and its role in the treatment of diabetes, no history would be complete without discussion of some of the controversy that arose after they published their findings.

Other medical scientists before Banting and Best had also succeeded in isolating a pancreatic secretion that alleviated the diabetic symptoms in experimental animals. Three scientists were definitely on the road to the application of insulin to humans, but for one reason or another were unable to use it clinically to demonstrate its effectiveness.

While N. C. Paulesco, a Rumanian physician, is frequently acknowledged as having isolated the hormone, which he called pancreine, and had demonstrated its effectiveness in diabetic dogs in 1916, it is also recognized that his work was preceded in 1908 by G. S. Zuelzer in Germany. Zuelzer's reports indicate clearly that he had an active but unpurified extract. He really was the first who dared to use it clinically, reporting its ameliorating effect on hyperglycemia, glycosuria, acetonemia, and acetonuria in several patients with decompensated diabetes. However, serious side effects forced him to discontinue his studies and cost him the support for a purification of the hormone.

Another investigator was an American named I. S. Kleiner, whose studies antedate even those of Paulesco's. He injected a filtrate of dog pancreas into depancreatized animals but was disturbed by reactions that now would be classified as insulin shock or insulin reaction. He therefore stopped his clinical applications until further purification of the substance could be achieved.

These three men, especially, deserve credit for their work, which preceded the final delivery of insulin by Banting and Best. No researcher works in a vacuum, and this is especially true in medicine, where reports in the medical literature are perused avidly by the profession. Discoveries and accomplishments in medicine must stand the test of scrutiny by scientific peers and must be reproducible by others who study the original data.

There is no doubt that Banting and Best built on previous work, but in 1921 the "fruit was ripe for picking" and they harvested it for the everlasting benefit of mankind. Beyond that, they were fortunate in having access to resources that resulted in improvement of the original product. A Rockefeller Fellow named J. B. Collip was assigned by Professor Macleod to the task of purifying enough insulin for large-scale clinical trials.

Banting and Best were also fortunate in stimulating the interest of the Eli Lilly Company, which offered its facilities to make insulin available in mass quantities. They evolved a method of purification that so improved both the purity and the scale of production that early in 1923 the supply of insulin was adequate to meet the requirements of those institutions selected to study its clinical use.

Banting and Macleod shared the Nobel Prize for Physiology and Medicine in 1923, and there was considerable dismay expressed in the scientific community over this selection. Medical scientists over the world expressed astonishment over the exclusion of Best and Collip, and considerable resentment was engendered in Rumania over the neglect of Paulesco's work. However, there appears little doubt, in retrospect, that the work of Banting and Best with all of the surrounding and subsequent circumstances was the master stroke that finally brought insulin into widespread use as the prime treatment for diabetes.

From that point, experimenters were able to move in directions that resulted in the extraction of insulin from the pancreases of hogs and bulls, ensuring an adequate supply of purified hormone with little or no side effects. Further work was required because the original insulin was short-acting and required up to four injections a day, with consequent inconvenience to the patient as well as the presence of the danger of infection from such liberal use of the hypodermic needle.

Discovery followed discovery as the search for longer-lasting insulin continued. Substances were found which, when combined with pure insulin, provided a steady and prolonged absorption of the hormone from a subcutaneous injection. This was accomplished in 1936 by D. H. C. Hagedorn and his associates in Denmark, and this, after the first extraction of insulin, was probably the most significant advance in diabetic management. Various types of insulin were developed—NPH, which acts promptly to lower the blood sugar but which persists for twenty-four hours; lente insulin, which has a slower first effect but also is long-lasting; and others. These newer insulin compounds enabled a diabetic to maintain what was thought to be reasonably good control with only one injection a day rather than three or four.

One of the prime characteristics of medical science that is fortunate for mankind is its absolute refusal to stand still. Even though an accomplishment or development may solve a medical problem or ameliorate a condition, almost immediately work is started to improve it still further.

So it was with diabetes. While the medical world accepted insulin as the treatment of choice and the main control factor in diabetes management, there were those who felt that if a drug could be found that could be taken orally and reduce the blood sugar, the treatment of the diabetic patient would be simplified. It was determined early in the insulin era that the hormone could not be taken by mouth, because the digestive enzymes in the stomach destroy it before it can pass into the bloodstream.

As another example of the serendipity that often occurs in research, a number of scientists who were looking for antibiotics noted hypoglycemic reactions in their laboratory animals. In 1948 R. Jonbon and A. L. Loubatiéres, of the Institute of Biology, Montpellier, France, who were experimenting with sulfa drugs to combat typhoid fever found that the rats with which they were working developed hypoglycemia after administration of one of their compounds. This led them down the road to application of the drug in diabetics, and it was found that the same condition obtained in human subjects.

Other people followed the same line of experimentation, and a number of drugs were found to have an effect on blood sugar when administered orally. Some worked well but produced toxic side effects; yet others were effective with no deleterious results. The latter have made their way into the medication resources of the physician managing certain diabetics because they are effective for the particular person. Some later studies by the University Group Diabetes Program flashed danger signals in the long-term employment of the oral agents, finding a higher incidence of heart disease among patients taking these drugs than in the normal population, or even in the diabetic population being treated with insulin alone. This has caused considerable discussion among diabetologists, which is still unresolved.

For many years physicians had considered that the sole hormone vital to control of diabetes was insulin; that the lack of this substance brought about the disease; and that by providing it through injection, diabetes could be brought under control. In 1950 this belief was severely jolted when Solomon Berson and Rosalyn Yalow developed a radioimmunoassay test that was able to make accurate determinations of the level of insulin in the blood. Utilizing the procedure, it was found that certain diabetics did have circulating insulin but showed all of the symptoms of diabetes. Others, notably those who had the disease from an early age, were found to have no insulin whatsoever.

As this is being written, scientists are reporting work that points toward multihormonal influences in the etiology of diabetes, as well as defects at various points in the cycle of insulin delivery to the cells where it performs its mission. No longer is diabetes being considered merely the result of insulin deficiency.

Thus modern-day scientists, while grateful that Banting and Best made their landmark contribution to the management of diabetes that has enabled many diabetics to live long and fruitful lives, now realize that the Canadian scientists did not really provide the total solution. And these same scientists are finding, as did the ancients and the middle-century people, that the more being discovered about diabetes, the more mysterious and complicated it is found to be. They now know that there is still a long way to go in accumulating the knowledge that eventually, it is hoped, will isolate the basic cause of the disease and thus point the way to its eventual eradication.

3

What Is Diabetes?

While the symptoms and manifestations of diabetes, as well as its clinical course in patients, have been known for more than three thousand years, exactly why it occurs and precisely how it acts is still a matter of considerable discussion, conjecture, and study.

The landmark studies of Von Mering and Minkowski decisively demonstrated that the organ fundamentally involved in the disease is the pancreas. Studies by Langerhans described the areas in the pancreas, the islets of Langerhans, that secreted the hormone that became known as insulin. More refined work isolated the secretion of insulin to the B, or Beta, cells in the islets. Then in 1921 came the final purification of an extract of these cells by Banting and Best, as insulin, and its application to diabetic patients with the result that the acute symptoms of diabetes could be controlled.

The progress following these discoveries gave rise to improvement in management techniques that have ameliorated the symptoms and enabled diabetics to live a reasonably normal life with a span approaching that of nondiabetics. However, little light has been shed on the underlying cause or causes of the disease, the fundamental defect or defects existing in the body that sooner or later evoke the appearance of diabetes.

It would be well at this point to define diabetes mellitus. Just what is it? It is a disease of unknown cause with a very important genetic element in its etiology. A major feature appears as an inability to metabolize carbohydrates normally, due either to impaired production of insulin or to a defect somewhere in the normal process of insulin activity. The carbohydrates, in the form of glucose, accumulate in the blood and because of their high concentration, overflow into the urine. As the disease progresses, abnormal carbohydrate metabolism becomes associated with additional derangement in the metabolism of fats and proteins.

In its severe form it is frequently called "insulin-dependent," "ketosis-prone," or "juvenile-onset" diabetes since it is the type most often seen in young people. In this manifestation the untreated disease may progress rapidly to a gravely imbalanced metabolic state, ketoacidosis, which can result in coma and death unless controlled by the administration of insulin. The less acute form of the disease is called "insulin-independent," "ketosis-resistant," or "maturity-onset" diabetes since it usually occurs later in life. Many cases of this form of the disease can be controlled by means other than insulin—weight reduction and limitation of carbohydrate intake, for example. Despite what seems to be proper control, in many cases progressive changes may occur in both juvenile- and maturity-onset diabetes that can lead to gradual deterioration of the blood vessels, the kidneys, the nervous system, and the vision (due to changes in the retina of the eye). Diabetes in children is still a rather rare situation when compared to the total population with the disease. However, the juvenile type, with its consequent requirement for insulin, can occur at any age.

The ability to provide insulin to diabetics, thereby controlling the disease, while beneficial in one sense—permitting patients to live longer and better—led medical science down the garden path to consider diabetes as being caused only by a deficiency of the hormone. So the accepted theory was that, by injecting insulin extracted from animal sources, the disease could be "cured."

The discovery that turned the conceptualization of the disease completely around, a work that should be considered another landmark in its history, was that some diabetics did have insulin in the bloodstream. When this was disclosed by Berson and Yalow in 1950 through their development of a radioimmunoassay method of accurately measuring circulating insulin, the realization dawned on medicine that perhaps there was more to diabetes than a simple deficiency of the hormone. Without going into the complex details of the technique, it indicated that a significant number of adult diabetics, instead of having no measurable insulin in their blood, had normal amounts and even in some cases an elevated amount when measured in the course of determining how sugar (glucose) is handled in the body. This reopened the entire field of investigation into the early changes in diabetes, and it focused attention on areas outside the pancreas as suspected of involvement in the development and course of diabetes.

Early studies following the development of radioimmunoassay demonstrated that insulin response to oral glucose loading in mild diabetes in adults was characterized by delayed secretion of the hormone, with a subsequent late rise in the insulin concentration to levels higher than those in nondiabetic subjects under similar conditions.

The situation was found to be somewhat different in youngsters with diabetes, where marked hyperglycemia was generally associated with little or no detectable insulin. It became obvious that the physiological mechanisms operative in the juvenile were very different from those in the adult diabetic. This was not fully appreciated until the radioimmunoassay technique was perfected. There is some difference of opinion among physicians about whether the high insulin concentration noted in the adult diabetic is truly as high as it appears. For H. S. Seltzer, Chief of Endocrinology Section, Veterans Administration Hospital, Dallas, Texas, is of the opinion that the insulin secretion in these patients is still inadequate considering the intensity of the stimulus of the blood glucose causing the response. Suffice it to say, however, that medical science now knows that there are two types of diabetics—those who secrete insulin and those who do not.

How, then, to explain that certain diabetics, namely those with adult-onset disease, have insulin in measurable amounts present in the blood and still are symptomatic? Consider the mechanism that operates to deliver insulin from its point of production to the areas where it is utilized. The normal sequence of events is as follows: the insulin is produced in the Beta cell in the islets of Langerhans and then is transported through the substance of the islets to the periphery of the pancreas, where it is released in small packets into the bloodstream. It is released not as insulin but in a large molecule called pro-insulin, which must be modified into active insulin. The end product is then carried in the bloodstream to the membranes of the many different cells, where it performs its assigned task of assisting in the metabolism of glucose, by attaching to the cell membrane and enabling the glucose to enter the cell. Its presence thus unlocks the cell door to glucose, which is metabolized inside the cell.

Therefore the defect that makes insulin less effective can be present at any one of these points in the process, and there are many opinions concerning which is the most important. There may be something faulty within the Beta cells, either in their mechanism or in their number, so that less insulin is produced than is required. It is obvious that in those people who suffer pancreatic destruction caused by infection, tumors or injury, or have surgical removal of the pancreas, diabetes develops because of the absolute loss of Beta cells. This is called "acquired" or "secondary" diabetes and, while they are not true diabetics genetically, they require injected insulin to survive.

There may be something awry in the system that moves the insulin from the Beta cell to the bloodstream. It is possible that a substance exists in the blood that destroys or inactivates the insulin, or that there is some factor tending to prevent the large pro-insulin molecule from being modified to active insulin. In addition, there may be something preventing the final insulin molecule from attaching to its normal receptor site on the cell, or there may be something faulty in the receptor sites, either in number or availability. Any or all of these would have the net effect of making insulin unable to play its designated role.

Some information about what actually does happen and what are the first changes can be obtained by studying the earliest stage in diabetes, called "prediabetes" or "potential diabetes." There is no simple test to determine the presence of prediabetes, and it is really a concept based on the inherited patterns of the disease. Although there is no clear agreement on the genetic laws governing the transmission of the diabetic trait or tendency, all investigators are convinced that the disease has a strong and undeniable basis in inheritance. It is known without a doubt that the incidence of diabetes is definitely higher in families that show diabetes in past generations than in families that show no history of the disease.

As regards prediabetes, it is convenient to think that the offspring of two diabetic parents, or the identical twin of a known diabetic, has the genetic tendency to become diabetic, and this is the individual considered to be prediabetic. The term does not mean undetected diabetes, and perhaps the better designation would be potential diabetic. Since it is only a suspicion, prediabetes cannot be diagnosed by procedures used in patient care. There is, in fact, even no assurance that an individual is prediabetic until a time when clinically recognizable diabetes is developed.

A firm diagnosis can be made only in retrospect. Prediabetes may begin with conception and last only a few years, as in the person who is afflicted with juvenile-onset disease, or it may continue for many years, as in those who develop maturity-onset diabetes. When prediabetics are tested with the common measures used to detect latent or unsuspected diabetes, their responses are completely normal. In fact, the only significant defect that has been noted in most of these people is the demonstration of a delay in the release of insulin in response to a glucose challenge, when insulin and glucose are determined in the same blood specimen. There have been other findings in prediabetics upon which there is truly no general agreement. These include a low level of certain blood proteins, decreases in the electrical activity of the retina of the eye, diminished amplitude of finger pulsation waves, higher levels of serum glucagon and changes in the structure of certain muscle membranes.

The presence of various abnormalities and specific substances peculiar to prediabetics could explain many of the features of diabetes that are still puzzling. This would be convenient were these to be found valid because physicians would then have a marker for diabetes that was not dependent upon changes in the blood sugar. It would be present were the patient eventually to have frank diabetes and absent if the opposite were true.

Overt diabetes seems to be the final outcome of the unsuccessful battle of the pancreas to compensate for its own shortcomings in insulin production, as well as its inability to overcome outside forces opposing the proper utilization of the hormone in carbohydrate metabolism.

Concerning pro-insulin and the possible problems surrounding its modification into the usable hormone, if it is only half as active as insulin in lowering blood sugar and an increase of pro-insulin is needed because of faulty conversion, the pancreas will produce large amounts in an attempt to keep the blood sugar normal. Therefore, in addition to a possible inherent defect in the Beta cell, it may be hyperreacting and exhausting itself in an attempt to produce a substance that then is not fully effective in lowering the blood sugar levels. This might account for the theory of Beta cell attenuation, which puts the blame for some of the defects in diabetes, not on the Beta cell itself, but on the conversion mechanism of pro-insulin.

An interesting theory again placing the blame within the Beta cell is that the diabetic is unable to regenerate Beta cells to replace those lost as a function of time or aging. Therefore, in this defect, the nature and cause of which is still unclear, the diabetic has less functioning insulin-producing units.

Another theory that places the defect outside of the Beta cell is that the diabetic may have a heightened resistance in the rest of the body's tissues to the action of insulin, so that increased amounts must be produced to achieve what would be a normal effect in a nondiabetic person. Therefore, the Beta cells must again work overtime and produce more insulin, becoming exhausted because of a defect in utilization in the periphery rather than because of any intrinsic defect within themselves. These two views—that there might be a conversion defect in pro-insulin, and the possibility of peripheral resistance to insulin as a cause of pancreatic exhaustion with the consequent occurrence of diabetes—are held in esteem by some investigators.

Putting together all the areas where the defect may lie in diabetes, the ability of the pancreas to produce insulin depends on the number of secretory units or Beta cells and on the rate at which the hormone can be made in response to a glucose challenge. It is probably genetically determined and can be described as the insulinogenic reserve. This is the basic situation that obtains in the pancreas and determines the pancreatic ability to cope with demand for insulin. In addition, if extrapancreatic factors existed to cause Beta cell exhaustion, normal carbohydrate metabolism will break down and the blood sugar level would increase to higher than normal.

What, then, could be some of these extrinsic precipitating diabetogenic factors that would cause a vulnerable pancreas finally to deteriorate and permit diabetes to occur? The first would be growth, which is a severe physiological stress situation. The second might be psychological or emotional stress, and the appearance of diabetes after great emotional tension following a divorce or the death of a family member has been noted for many years. The process through which stress may work might be the increased activity of cortisone or adrenalin, or through some cerebral mechanism that tips the balance in favor of pancreatic failure. The third would be infection, which causes an increase in metabolic activity that the pancreas may not be able to meet.

Other endocrine diseases such as adrenal or thyroid dysfunction might bring on diabetes. Another situation would be pregnancy, which causes emotional as well as physiological stress in some women, intensifying the metabolic needs for which an inadequate pancreas may not be able to provide. The process of aging in itself is a strong causative factor in a genetically primed individual.

The final factor, which has probably received the most attention as a diabetogenic cause, is obesity. It is known that the majority of maturity-onset diabetics are overweight, and it may be that the fatter body cells of obese individuals actually require more insulin to help transport glucose into the cell than those of thinner individuals. Insulin acts at the cell membrane, mediating the movement of glucose into the body cells, where it is metabolized into the energy required for the cell activity. If extra insulin is required because of obesity's effect at the cell membrane level, the secretory activity of the pancreas may become drained. Thus, if there is an inherent pancreatic defect, the heightened demand may cause exhaustion of the Beta cell after a period of time.

Experiments have shown that the fasting insulin level tends to increase linearly with body weight, independent of the presence of diabetes. This would tend to bear out the conclusion that more insulin is required in obese individuals than in lean persons. In the normal individual the base-line level of insulin response shows that, when needed, the basic insulin secretion is increased and the ability of the Beta cell to produce more insulin is also increased. In diabetics, where there is carbohydrate intolerance without obesity, the base-line level may be normal but there is a poor response to a glucose load. In diabetics with obesity there seems to be an increase in the base-line level of insulin but a diminished responsiveness. This has brought up the possibility of a dissociation between basic insulin secretion and the responsiveness of the Beta cells to stimuli. There may well be two Beta cell activities, one that releases constantly to produce base-line secretion, and the other for quick release and heightened production in response to glucose challenges.

It would seem, therefore, that there are three independent factors that must interplay and function to produce diabetes. The first, which seems to be fundamental to the genesis of the disease, is that an intrinsic weakness exists in the Beta cells. To this should be added some extrapancreatic diabetogenic elements, which are still in question and which may involve increased resistance at the cellular level, or defects in the conversion of pro-insulin to insulin. Further, there may appear in the tissues or the blood some substances destructive of insulin or inhibitory to its proper action. The final stimulating factor required would be one that pushes the pancreas to or beyond the limits of its capabilities.

All of these things can combine to cause a diminution of pancreatic activity resulting in a level of insulin production that is no longer adequate to contain the blood sugar within normal limits.

The hypothesis that diabetes is a bihormonal disorder and not merely a simple lack of insulin has been reinforced in recent years by studies of the action of glucagon, a substance manufactured by the Alpha cells in the pancreas. Oddly enough, the hormone was recognized in 1923, only two years after insulin was first used in the treatment of diabetes, but was considered to be only a contaminant of insulin, to be extracted in the purification process. In the early insulin preparations it was identified as the substance causing an unexpected rise in blood sugar after injection of insulin. Glucagon and insulin are adversaries—glucagon raises blood glucose, insulin lowers it; and each has an opposite effect on other metabolic processes.

Recent research reported by Dr. Roger H. Unger of the University of Texas Southwestern Medical School in Dallas has suggested that diabetic hyperglycemia may result from a lack of insulin coupled with an excess of glucagon, rather than from insulin deficiency alone.

Now in the early stages of research is the activity of a small protein isolated from the brain, called somatostatin, with which experimenters have suppressed glucagon activity. Originally, when it was extracted from the hypothalamus, somatostatin was found to inhibit the release of growth hormone from the pituitary gland, but it was also found to depress the release of both glucagon and insulin. Its ultimate effect and possible use in diabetes is being studied extensively and may prove valuable in management of the disease.

It is interesting to speculate on the role played by infection in diabetes, specifically regarding further insults to the pancreas. It is known that the mumps virus, as well as other virus types, will definitely affect the pancreas. Diabetes has been observed in animal colonies where viral infection was introduced into one member, causing diabetes, and then almost the entire colony developed the disease. So viral infection as a factor affecting the intrinsic pancreatic activity is receiving a considerable amount of attention in the study of the causes of diabetes.

It is readily seen that diabetes is more easily described in terms of its symptoms and course than in definition of its cause. A genetic basis, true, but where exactly is the defect that is transmitted? The inheritable aspect must be recognized as basic because the other influences that have been described as diabetogenic are present in most of the population, who do not ever become afflicted with the disease. All fat people do not acquire the disease, nor do all pregnant women or people who go through severe emotional stress or those who suffer endocrine disorders. So the common factor must be hereditary in all of those who become diabetic, no matter what the precipitating factors. As the science of genetics becomes increasingly knowledgeable, perhaps the future will reveal enough information to shed more light on diabetes, as well as on other diseases that are also recognized to possess a fundamental hereditary characteristic.

4

Are You a Diabetic?

Compared to defining precisely what diabetes is, the decision concerning who is a diabetic is relatively simple. A diagnosis of diabetes is made upon the determination of an error in metabolism disclosed by tests indicating the presence in the blood of an abnormally high amount of glucose, which is the simplest form of sugar.

The foodstuffs the body uses are divided into three main types: carbohydrates, fats, and proteins. Carbohydrates are found in potatoes, rice, and bread products, as well as in milk, fruits, and vegetables. The metabolism of these substances produces glucose, which is delivered to all portions of the body by means of the bloodstream. Since the brain uses glucose very extensively in its function, a certain amount of it is necessary at all times, since a lack can result in irreversible brain damage. Therefore, even under conditions of extreme food deprivation, the body tries to ensure the presence of glucose to some degree even if it must be derived from other food sources. Protein can form sugar in the course of its metabolism, if needed.

Then what does it mean when the diabetic has too much sugar in the blood?

The nondiabetic individual is able to maintain the levels of his blood sugar between relatively narrow limits whether he is in a fasting or fed state. Even after a meal rich in carbohydrate, the normal individual will rarely show a blood sugar higher than 160 milligrams percent (mg%), and even in periods of extreme starvation the sugar level will rarely fall below 60 mg%. The nondiabetic is able to stabilize the blood sugar because the pancreas responds to the stimulus of glucose by releasing insulin quickly and in an appropriate amount. The insulin brings about a lowering of the blood sugar by facilitating its transport into the various cells, where it is metabolized to furnish energy for body functions.

The diabetic, unfortunately, is unable to maintain this fine control of the blood sugar. The blood sugar cannot be kept within certain acceptable limits either in response to the ingestion of sugar or, sometimes, in the fasting state. This is in keeping with the classical definition of diabetes as a disease where the blood sugar rises to excessive heights in response to a sugar load, or may do so even in a fasting situation. Said another way, the diabetic cannot keep his blood sugar under control in the face of stresses and strains of eating, fasting, emotional disturbances, infection, exercise, and the use of certain medications. Because the sugar is not being metabolized properly, owing to a defect in the insulin mechanism, it accumulates in the blood and spills over into the urine. The excess of sugar in the blood may cause changes in many organs of the body, ranging from the blood vessels to the eyes.

All diabetics by definition must have instability of their

blood sugar when measured under various circumstances. The clinical expression, the picture of diabetes, can vary from being very mild or latent with virtually no symptoms to manifesting itself as a very intense and ferocious disease. Similarly, the laboratory tests for diabetes may also show this variation of intensity.

This may well be illustrated by several examples at various points in the spectrum of diabetes.

A fifty-year-old man goes to his physician for an annual checkup. He is feeling quite well, although complaining of a bit of chronic fatigue, but showing no other symptoms that even his local newsstand dealer or a nosy neighbor would deduce as being suggestive of diabetes. He is, however, twenty pounds overweight, and his medical history reveals that a maternal grandmother had diabetes. The examination is completely negative and normal, with no sugar appearing in the urine. His physician is a rather astute observer, though, and because the patient is over the age of forty-five, is obese, and has a positive family history, he orders a postprandial (after-eating) sugar test. This differs from the fasting blood sugar test in that a sugar load is given to challenge the insulin-glucose relationship. In this case the patient's blood sugar measured 220 mg% after two hours, clearly in the abnormal range and clearly consistent with the diagnosis of diabetes.

A somewhat different example is that of a ten-year-old child who develops a sore throat, becomes progressively sicker, begins vomiting, runs a high fever, is listless, and then becomes nearly comatose. When taken to a hospital emergency room, the youngster goes into a coma, breathing rapidly and shallowly. An appropriate series of examinations reveals a blood sugar of 500 mg% and various substances called acetone and ketone bodies in the urine, and the little patient is found to be in a state of ketoacidosis, which is the most severe, ferocious, and violent expression of diabetes. In this situation, no other testing is needed to uncover the metabolic abnormality of diabetes; it is apparent right at the outset.

In another case, a female patient, aged fifty-six, came to the physician with a large boil on her face, which was opened and cleaned out, then healed rather slowly. Otherwise the patient, who was 5 feet 6 inches tall and weighed 190 pounds, felt perfectly well and had no other untoward symptoms except some vaginal itching. Her mother had been diagnosed as diabetic two weeks previously, so the physician suggested a blood sugar test. It showed 300 mg% of sugar in the blood, obviously in the diabetic category.

A forty-year-old patient who was feeling well noted that his vision was blurry, with the eyes not quite focusing. His ophthalmologist found a great change in vision, but otherwise the patient seemed in good health. The spectacles that were prescribed improved the vision for a few weeks and then appeared to provide no help whatsoever. When the patient was referred to his physician for a complete checkup, his medical history elicited the facts that he had lost five pounds in the previous month, was thirstier than usual, and was getting up to urinate two or three times each night whereas before he had been sleeping right through. Tests found sugar in the urine and a blood sugar of 250 mg%. The changing visual acuity was due to variations in the body's fluid balance, which modified the shape of the eyes and caused sight difficulties. The combination of symptoms with the results of the blood tests indicated definitely that the patient was diabetic.

A twenty-five-year-old bachelor and man-about-town who prided himself on his sexual prowess noted with a great deal of distress a diminution in libido and some difficulty in achieving an erection. His physician found the fasting blood sugar normal, but because of a family history of diabetes did other, more intensive tests that indicated a blood sugar of 300 mg%. The diagnosis was diabetes with impotence as an early manifestation.

A forty-year-old woman had recently divorced her husband, who was having an affair. The court proceedings were hectic and bitter, with many recriminatory accusations exchanged over custody of the children and the amount of alimony. Two weeks after the climax of the court arguments and its corollary distress she began to have itching in various parts of her body, became inordinately thirsty, and started to urinate very frequently. She became progressively more fatigued, lethargic, and barely able to stand up. She was taken to a hospital and tests indicated a blood sugar of 400 mg%, with ketone bodies and acetone in the urine. She was admitted immediately to the intensive care unit with a diagnosis of diabetic coma with ketoacidosis, probably precipitated by severe emotional stress.

Thus it is readily seen that there are manifestations of the disease at extreme ends of the spectrum of symptoms, as well as infinite variations in between. The two most diametrically opposed forms of diabetes are that of juvenile-onset and that of maturity-onset, expressed in a gentler, more benign fashion and with lesser effect than that found in juveniles, where its course is rapid, violent, and explosive so that if treatment is not begun almost immediately, the results will be dire indeed.

Where, then, does one look most carefully to detect diabetes? Obviously, it would be impractical to put everyone in the United States through the ritual of a complicated glucose challenge test, so it would be most productive to cover the population at highest risk. And who are these people? They are those who possess characteristics similar to the ones discussed in the previous chapters on the factors that may precipitate diabetes. Suspicion falls first on people who have a family history of the disease, on those over the age of forty, and on the obese. With the available clinical facilities at present, the diagnosis of diabetes depends on the demonstration of abnormal sugar metabolism. This should be done by means of a blood sugar test, because if the determination is made merely through the measurement of sugar in the urine, only the tip of the iceberg is revealed. Sugar does not spill over into the urine until the level in the blood exceeds about 170 mg%, so it is possible to have diabetes with blood sugars above normal but below the point at which the kidney excretes sugar into the urine. This is called the renal threshold for sugar. However, in certain patients, especially those who are older, this can vary tremendously and it is possible to have blood sugars of 200 mg%, 300 mg%, or even 400 mg% with no sugar evident in the urine. This can engender a false sense of security and a mistaken indication of good control, should only the urine sugar level be tested. It is essential to test the level of the sugar in the blood at stated intervals to make an exact determination concerning the state of control under which the patient is functioning.

On the question of obesity, there is no doubt that most maturity-onset diabetics are overweight. However, some patients lose weight when diabetes begins. They are the ones who have a significant amount of sugar in the urine. Normally no sugar is excreted in the urine, except in pregnancy and in some individuals who will tend to spill a little after very high carbohydrate meals. A diabetic who is not controlled can lose several hundred calories a day of unutilized sugar through the urine. Therefore, if an individual is eating 1,500 calories a day and keeping his weight steady, then loses 300 to 400 calories in his urine, he is effectively ingesting 1,200 calories, which in most people will cause weight reduction. Some diabetics who develop the presence of ketone bodies when their condition is detected, will lose the desire to eat because of the appetite-destroying effect of these substances.

If a fasting blood sugar is done, only a certain percentage of diabetics will show abnormalities. As a test, it does indicate a severe problem, though, because fasting sugars are usually taken twelve hours after the last meal and a high reading indicates that the body's mechanisms were unable to reduce the blood sugar to normal levels even in that period of time. But when the index of suspicion is high, the physician is not satisfied with either a urine sugar test or a fasting sugar determination. He does a postprandial sugar test where the stress of a sugar intake is placed on the individual. If the postprandial test is in any way doubtful or borderline, then a glucose tolerance test is ordered. This is a highly ritualized and standardized procedure in which a measured amount of glucose drink is given and blood is drawn at specific times to determine how the sugar is being metabolized. Then this is compared to the nondiabetic pattern, and the physician can see whether the patient responds as does a nondiabetic or, by being unable to dispose of the excess sugar, falls into the diabetic classification.

Since the glucose tolerance test is the main diagnostic tool in the determination of diabetes, it should be understood that the administration and interpretation of the test is not as simple and straightforward as described. There are factors involving age, preexisting diet, activity, and concurrent medication that can cause certain variations in results. It has been found that a morning test will give lower readings than one performed in the afternoon or evening. To ensure that insulin response will not be sluggish due to a low previous demand, the patient should consume a high carbohydrate diet for three days prior to the test. Since fever and infection distort the GTT results, it is inaccurate to do the test when signs or symptoms of these conditions are present. Also, the GTT curve has been shown to vary with age, changing with each decade of life, so that data that would be indicative of diabetes in a younger patient may not mean the same thing in an older one. These are general guidelines, and it falls to the physician to interpret the test patterns for the patient.

Yet, while all diabetics are hyperglycemic, showing high blood sugars in various tests, not all hyperglycemia is diabetic in origin. Many physicians specializing in the care of diabetics will see cases where the hyperglycemia has come and gone—in a female during pregnancy, or in a susceptible person, male or female, following a period of inactivity and overeating, or under the stress of disease. The World Health Organization Expert Committee on Diabetes Mellitus in the report of its meeting in 1964 recommended that the following definitions of diabetes mellitus and related states be adopted as standard throughout the medical profession. These are:

POTENTIAL DIABETICS
> Persons in whom diabetes may be predicted with reasonable accuracy. While they may respond normally to a GTT, there is a clear risk of their developing diabetes. They include:
> The identical twin of a diabetic;
> A person whose parents were both diabetic;
> A person with one diabetic parent whose other, although nondiabetic, has or had a diabetic parent, sibling, or off-spring, or a sibling with a diabetic child;
> A woman who has born a live or stillborn child weighing more than nine pounds.

LATENT DIABETICS
> (1) A person in whom the GTT is normal but who has a history of a diabetic GTT at some time—during pregnancy, during infection, under stress, or when overweight.
> (2) A person who has abnormal blood glucose responses such as those found in diabetes in intensified tests such as the cortisone-augmented GTT.

ASYMPTOMATIC (SUBCLINICAL OR CHEMICAL) DIABETICS
> (1) A person with a diabetic response to the GTT whose fasting blood sugar is below 130 mg%.
> (2) As above, but with fasting blood sugars above normal values.

CLINICAL DIABETIC
> A person with an abnormal response to the GTT or an increased fasting blood sugar and with the complications or symptoms of diabetes.

Since the entire diagnosis of diabetes hinges on the demonstration of glucose abnormality, which may be borderline or not always absolutely clear, an improved means of determination based on other factors would be of inestimable value.

For example, if someone at the age of forty-five started to show sugar in the urine and at the point was diagnosed as diabetic, the genetic tendency for the disease was probably present. Therefore, if this forty-five-year-old had had a GTT ten years previously, diabetes might have been diagnosed at that time. And had an even more sensitive type of GTT (with cortisone) been given at age twenty, the diagnosis might have been made then.

What physicians would really appreciate having is the ability to diagnose diabetes almost at birth, when the genetic tendency is present but at a time far in advance of the development of abnormalities in glucose metabolism. If this could be done, those people who in later life might or would become diabetic could be identified and steps possibly could be taken to prevent the occurrence of the disease. By treating these people early with diet control that might prevent exhaustion of the Beta cells, the onset of glucose metabolism abnormalities might be averted, as well as the degenerative changes common in long-term frank diabetes.

Actually, the great need in the diagnostic technique in diabetes is for the identification of a genetic or other marker. This would be the discovery of a characteristic that is not dependent on glucose abnormalities but that would indicate whether or not the individual under study possessed the genetic tendency for diabetes. There have been various attempts at finding such a marker—the presence of an albumin antagonist to insulin, called synalbumin; the discovery of zinc excretion of high degree in the urine of potential diabetics; the investigation of cell structure changes such as basement membrane thickening; and the presence of abnormal hemoglobin in those people thought to be prediabetic.

Of these, two have captured the imagination of physicians: the presence of synalbumin, which was thought to block the action of insulin; and basement membrane thickening. The man who first propounded the theory of synalbumin and its action was Dr. John Vallance-Owens, professor of medicine at Queens University in Belfast, Ireland. In 1958 he reported that he had found in the blood of diabetics that serum albumin had the property of inactivating insulin, and he proposed this as a means of determining prediabetes without reference to glucose. He published this work in 1961, and then in 1962 he made animals diabetic and found that the synalbumin was not a genetic marker for the disease but differentiated true diabetes from experimentally induced diabetes. Other researchers were unable to reproduce his results, and it was realized some years later that the equipment used by Vallance-Owens was not described correctly, so other scientists could not match his work. However, in 1972 and 1973 George N. Holcomb and William E. Dulin of the diabetes research division of the Upjohn Company performed the experiments and showed that Vallance-Owens was correct in his description of the action of synalbumin. But it still does not appear that this was definitive and could serve by its presence to predict the advent of diabetes.

Dr. Marvin Siperstein, of the University of California in San Francisco, has described the thickening of tissue basement membranes as being significantly greater in prediabetics than in normal people. He found basement membrane thickening in mid-thigh muscle capillaries in 8 percent of nondiabetics, 74 percent of prediabetics, and 98 percent of overt diabetics. Among his conclusions were that basement membrane thickening is found in most human diabetics and that it is not affected by the duration or severity of the disease. He also concluded that induced diabetes in animals is not accompanied by basement membrane thickening. According to Siperstein, diabetes may result from basement membrane thickening in the pancreas that interferes with the proper functioning of the insulin production and delivery system.

But others—Joseph Williamson and Charles Kilo of the Washington University School of Medicine in St. Louis— have drawn other conclusions. They take issue with Siperstein's technique of measurement and the area of the body he chose. They found that the more dependent vessels, even in nondiabetics, tended to have basement membrane thickening. They then went to the St. Louis Zoo and measured basement membranes of a giraffe's neck, finding that the lower on the neck the area tested was, the thicker the basement membrane, so they concluded that the thickening was due to gravitational pressure above the point tested. This was also done in people, and they found less thickening in the deltoid muscle of the shoulder than in the calf of the leg. Aging was also a factor—older people tended to have thicker basement membrane than did younger ones.

At this time, none of the so-called markers has survived under intensive investigation, and people are still looking for the elusive clues to indicate a diagnosis of diabetes unquestionably, before the glucose abnormalities appear. Just about the only thing on which there is agreement is that there is some disorder and delay of insulin release in the prediabetic. What it is and why and how it begins are wide open to question and investigation. A simple clinical means for marking and recognizing the prediabetic would help perhaps in preventing or delaying the onset of overt diabetes. On the other side of the coin, if a patient with a predisposing genetic background was found, through use of a marker, not to be prediabetic or a potential diabetic, he would not have to worry about coming down with the disease later in life.

Since none of the markers has proved valid beyond a doubt, the physician must rely on good history-taking, a high degree of suspicion, and the use of appropriate glucose studies and glucose tolerance tests to diagnose diabetes. At present, diabetes is defined in terms of its own definition. Diabetes is said to exist when there is a blood sugar higher than normal, with perhaps sugar showing in the urine. Thus diabetes is diagnosed as the patient's having intolerance to glucose because the tests show he has intolerance to glucose. This is like saying that a patient has had a coronary attack because he has had a closure of one of the major blood vessels supplying the heart muscle. It is also like saying that one is John Smith because one's name is John Smith.

It is possible to say that a person has had a coronary attack because he had chest pain, alterations in the results of certain blood tests, and disturbances in his electrocardiograms compatible with the other findings. All these symptoms mean that there has been a closure of one of the vessels in the heart that has killed some heart muscle, and what is seen is the heart muscle damage. Therefore a coronary attack has occurred.

It is not possible, on the other hand, to say this about diabetes at this time. All that can be said is that a patient has diabetes because his blood sugar is behaving in an abnormal manner. It cannot be said that the disease is present because the pancreas is releasing insulin poorly or that the insulin it is releasing is not being utilized properly owing to the action of any one of a number of factors. These facts may be true, but they cannot be clearly delineated in a clinical situation now. The test for insulin in the blood is still only a research tool, not in everyday practical use, for employment in studies of insulin secretion and release. The hope for the future is that the measurement of insulin response to glucose challenge by means of ultrasensitive tests may lead to early detection of diabetes more accurately than do any of the present means.

As the disease itself is unfathomed in its cause and mysterious in its action, it is equally so in the way it strikes. There are an infinite variety and combinations of triggering mechanisms that can set off the diabetes explosion, and it is not possible to predict accurately where and when it will occur in a particular individual. Only one factor seems to be something of a common denominator—the genetic tendency. This can be suspected only where there is a family history of the disease and does not always hold true because of the manner in which the laws of heredity operate. The disease skips a generation now and then and may cause diabetes to appear in one descendant while ignoring others in the same family.

There is considerable merit, though, in evaluating the family history early in life to disclose the genetic tendency. Accepting the fact that a young child whose family tree contains diabetes may at some time become diabetic should influence its life-style, especially as pertains to diet and the prevention of obesity. While it may not always be possible to prevent the disease, perhaps its onset can be delayed for a number of years so that its course is shorter and less destructive in the ultimate complications that may follow. Until the discovery of a sign that definitely predicts diabetes, this might be a prudent road to follow.

5

Diet and Diabetes

Food has been a major concern of mankind since our earliest days on Earth. Fierce and bloody wars have been fought over the rights to hunt in particular areas, and early man earned the respect of his fellows by his ability to go into the forest and return with succulent items of nourishment for his family or tribe. The accolades "great warrior" and "great or mighty hunter" were equal in importance. Early man's instincts provided the knowledge that survival depended upon a continuing supply of nutritious material. Ancient nomadic peoples were essentially wanderers in search of sources of food for themselves and their flocks of domestic animals. It was only when they discovered that food could be grown in the ground, thus permitting them to remain in one place, that there developed a stable, static population, laying claim to parcels of acreage and creating town and village centers surrounded by their fertile fields.

Diet not only fills a physiological need but also is essential to psychological health. The kind of food eaten sometimes demonstrates and provides status. It furnishes mental satisfaction. It is important in social intercourse, and in ancient days if one "broke bread" with another, the process in effect guaranteed that peace would reign between the participants. Interestingly enough, *Roget's Thesaurus* gives as synonyms for "food" the phrases "good cheer" and "good living." The psychic satisfactions derived from food are considered so important that some physicians recommend that a strict reducing diet not be started while a person is in a psychological stress situation lest emotional damage be done because of food deprivation. And it is known that the desire for food when one is disturbed or worried transcends true hunger and metabolic need.

What could be more logical then that physicians through the centuries should turn to diet in search of cures for illnesses and diseases, even though those in ancient times knew little of the biochemical and metabolic reasons therefor? They noticed, undoubtedly, that along with an indisposition their patients suffered some change in appetite. They also must have observed that animals modified their diets when ill. The dog with an upset stomach, for example, will eat grass to provide a crude sort of cathartic to rid the gastrointestinal tract of offending material. The early physicians even evaluated the difference in a patient's progress when he ate lightly or heavily while sick. So, on no truly scientific basis and with little or no specific medication available, the ancients recommended diet modifications in various illnesses.

Thus it was eminently reasonable for the early physicians, and many in the Middle Ages and later, to have turned to diet as a means of controlling or curing diabetes. Despite their ignorance of body chemistry in general and metabolism in particular, they did feel that nutrition was an important treatment. Areteaus, who had provided the earliest complete description of diabetes, thought that milk, cereals, starches, autumn fruits, and sweet wine would be beneficial.

Later on, physicians occupied with the problems of diabetes came close to determining dietetic content that might be helpful. It must be remembered that before the discovery of insulin in 1921 there was really no effective treatment for the acute, severely symptomatic diabetic. There is every reason to believe that patients existed during earlier days, even as there are today, who had undetected diabetes or the disease with very mild symptoms, who lived normally until they became ill with the difficulties now known as the complications of diabetes.

But the overt diabetic, prior to insulin, had no recourse available to him other than diet. In 1796 Dr. John Rollo offered an approach to treatment through nutrition. Even though the basic food elements—carbohydrates, fats, and proteins—were not identified at the time, Rollo proposed a regimen low in carbohydrate and high in protein. This consisted mainly of suet pudding, milk, and pork.

Then in the late 1800s various schemes were suggested, all involving some sort of near-starvation or attempts to compensate for the drastic loss of sugar by prescribing a great deal of candy or even by having the patient drink his own urine.

In 1897 severe restrictive measures and alternate fast days became widely popular, but these were eventually replaced by the F. M. Allen regime, which came into prominence in 1914. This required careful preparation in the cooking of meals, with rigorous caloric control and carbohydrate limitation. The method included putting the patient on several days of actual starvation until the blood sugar fell to normal, then prescribing a diet containing less than 20 grams of carbohydrate per day. This treatment was successful in some cases of diabetes but failed in the more severe forms of the disease. From 1897 until 1914 the average length of life of all diabetics after detection of the disease was 4.9 years.

From 1914 until 1922 the average life-span was 6.1 years. Statistically, therefore, the Allen regime did seem to increase slightly the diabetic's chances of survival when compared to the results of treatment modes available in the decade or two prior to its use.

However, with the discovery of insulin, dietary therapy was relegated to a much less important role, often to the point of some neglect. The basic and vital importance of dietary management in the treatment of diabetes is frequently overlooked in this era of therapeutic enthusiasm and technological wizardry.

At a conference on endocrinology sponsored by the University of Chicago Pritzker School of Medicine in 1975, Dr. David Horwitz of the school's faculty said that dietary management should be the mainstay of diabetes therapy. Even when dietary management must be combined with insulin therapy, diet is important, since insulin "doesn't follow the food, food must follow the insulin." In his report Dr. Horwitz also stated that it is best to think about diet in terms of the natural history of diabetes and the history of the Beta cells. At birth, Beta cell integrity might be assumed to be 100 percent, with a gradual decline throughout life. In the normal individual the Beta cell reserve, despite some loss, remains within the range in which the individual will still be able to produce enough insulin to meet metabolic needs.

In the maturity-onset diabetic, this decline seems to come faster. Often metabolic demands can be kept below the theoretical threshold by spreading out food throughout the day to maintain normal carbohydrate metabolism.

As reported by *Internal Medicine News,* Dr. Horwitz continued by saying that the juvenile diabetic cannot be treated by dietary manipulation alone. His decline in Beta cell reserve occurs very fast, but some patients do have some Beta cell function for some time, with even a brief recovery period, the so-called "honeymoon" phase of diabetes.

Since obesity and associated insulin resistance increase

insulin demand, control of total caloric intake to attain ideal body weight is the single most important objective in dietary treatment of diabetes. According to the National Commission on Diabetes, the chance of developing diabetes doubles with every 20 percent of an individual's excess weight.

The ideal weight value can be obtained from any number of accepted sources such as nutrition textbooks or insurance company tables. As a rough guide, in women these tables usually allow 100 pounds for the first 5 feet of height and 5 pounds per inch thereafter; in men this would be changed to 120 pounds for the first 5 feet and 5 pounds per inch above that. These standards apply to people with medium frames, so for slightly or heavily built people 10 percent can be added or subtracted, depending on the estimate. The daily caloric requirement is approximately 10 times the ideal weight, but this can be refined slightly by reducing it 100 or 200 calories if the patient is over fifty years of age or is female. A crude appraisal must then be made of the additional caloric requirement in a patient, based on normal daily activities, to arrive at a figure for the ideal total daily caloric intake. This will usually be considerably below what the obese patient has actually been ingesting. In overweight diabetics, reducing the caloric intake and thus the weight will often bring about a lowering of the fasting blood sugar and even the reversal of an abnormal result on a glucose tolerance test.

The first question to be considered is whether or not dietary modification is necessary in all patients with diabetes. Although the subject is certainly controversial, it would seem that if a patient were at ideal weight and in good control—however this is measured—with no increase in blood fats and cholesterol, there would appear to be no compulsion to manipulate the diet. Unfortunately, this state of affairs obtains in only a small percentage of patients. The majority are either over- or undernourished, and it is these people for whom nutritional adjustments must be made.

However, it is easier in word than in deed to bring about

the reduction in weight in patients, diabetic or otherwise. The great American preoccupation with weight is expressed usually by "I have to take a little weight off, guess I'll go on a diet starting tomorrow." But tomorrow rarely arrives! Intake in some people has little to do with metabolic need. Certain foods seem to have a social status value, both in type and amount, and sometimes the obesity of one's spouse is an index of material success in the eyes of the community. It is easy to remember the day when a fat child was considered to be a healthy child. These factors, plus some that are beginning to be evaluated in sophisticated physiological and psychological experiments, tend to make strict adherence to a weight reduction schedule difficult for doctors and patients alike.

In the diabetic who is undernourished and taking insulin, dietary demands must be less casual than merely trying to have the patient attain ideal weight. These patients have special nutritional needs because of their metabolic abnormalities and lack of insulin of their own, but they, too, must maintain optimum weight.

Although the discovery and availability of insulin did tend to push dietary management in diabetes aside somewhat, the other side of the coin is that it also permitted less restriction in the diet so that more adequate nutrition could ensue. In the juvenile-onset diabetic it has meant being able to eat more normally, with a choice of foods more closely resembling those chosen by his peers—a very important factor psychologically. And the maturity-onset diabetic can hew to a regime more to his liking, which provides him with the energy necessary to do a normal day's work and to participate socially as well.

Prescribing a dietary regime that is acceptable to the diabetic in his daily round of activity certainly would go a long way toward lightening the unremitting burden of his chronic condition, making him less of a curiosity. This is especially true in children, who want desperately to be "one of the gang" in all respects. Since one aim of treatment is to maintain the patient in a happy, well-adjusted frame of mind, dining the way his social circle and family does is one means that should not be neglected.

What does "adequate nutrition" mean? Obviously, the body needs a balance in the major categories of foodstuffs—protein, carbohydrate, and fat. The concepts of how much of each is needed daily to provide a balanced diet change from time to time, but there is unanimity of opinion that all are required in some proportion. The physician who treats diabetics must individualize the dietary prescription so that the food intake is therapeutic for each particular patient.

As concerns the need for specific calorie amounts, some years ago the American Diabetes Association, together with the American Dietetic Association and the United States Public Health Service, published their joint opinion covering the daily caloric requirements of adult diabetic patients. Those who were overweight and under 5 feet 6 inches in height, if sedentary, should not exceed 1,200–1,500; if moderately active, 1,800; and very active, 2,200. Those already at desired weight and under 5 feet 6 inches, when sedentary should not exceed 1,800, when moderately active, 2,600, and very active, 3,000.*

In juveniles, according to Dr. Milton B. Handelsman of the State University of New York, Downstate Medical Center, writing in *Clinical Diabetes Mellitus* (edited by Dr. Max Ellenberg of the Mount Sinai School of Medicine in New York City and Dr. Harold Rifkin of the Albert Einstein College of Medicine), normal nutrition should be prescribed and adequate insulin dosage be given to ensure proper utilization of the ingested food.

A number of formulas have been used as guides for the proper caloric requirements in children. One uses height as a standard and recommends 35 calories per inch. Another uses

---

* For those above 5 feet 6 inches, the physician's appraisal of caloric need, based on activity and height, must be the guide.

weight and sets the need at 100 calories per kilogram (kg. = 2.2 pounds) at one year of age; 80 calories per kg. at age 5; 60 calories per kg. at age 10; 40 calories per kg. at age 15. Yet another formula uses age as a benchmark: 1,000 calories per day at one year, with an additional 100 calories for each succeeding year up to 13 for girls and 19 for boys. However, another factor must be taken into account in all dietary prescriptions—satiety, which is most important in obtaining cooperation on the part of the patient. If the diet leaves the person hungry and dissatisfied, it will not be followed.

A patient who weighs 180, who is diabetic, and whose ideal weight because of height and age should be 150 pounds needs a reducing diet, according to his physician. Thus, a 1,500-calorie-a-day regime is mapped out to bring him down to ideal weight. The diet, balanced as to components, would consist of 150 grams of carbohydrate for 600 calories, 70 grams of protein for 280 calories, and 70 grams of fat for 620 calories.

The diet is created for each individual as his metabolic requirements are evaluated. As far as protein is concerned, usually a total of one gram (4 calories) per day per kilogram of weight is sufficient. Patients who may be losing some protein in the urine because of associated kidney disease, or patients with intestinal absorption difficulties, may need more than this amount. A rough guide to the amount of carbohydrate allowance per day is to divide the total caloric requirement by 10, expressing the result in grams, at 4 calories per gram. It seems advantageous to make up the bulk of carbohydrate with the more slowly digested complex starches rather than the rapidly absorbed sugars. This tends to reduce wide swings in the blood sugar level. To restrict the carbohydrate intake below 120 grams per day is difficult from a practical standpoint, although it certainly can be done. There has been a considerable amount of discussion lately about the necessity for severe carbohydrate limitation in all diabetics and, indeed, whether diabetics who are given a freer reign in carbo-hydrate intake may in fact demonstrate more stability and a better degree of control than those in whom it is more rigidly limited.

Once the protein and carbohydrate components of the diet have been determined, the remainder consists of fat, at 9 cal-ories per gram. Since most diets that keep the carbohydrates down tend to increase the fat content, a potential problem arises because of the propensity of diabetics to atherosclerotic disease. There has been considerable argument over the amount of fats in the diet and whether these should be satu-rated or unsaturated. It is difficult to make an unequivocal statement about this at the present time. Basically, it depends on the opinion of the physician who is treating the patient. If the physician is convinced that a real or potentially abnormal lipid (fat) pattern can or should be corrected, then it is per-fectly within reason to substitute—not add—unsaturated fat for half the animal fat in the diet. If, on the other hand, the physician is not convinced that dietary fat is playing a role in blood vessel damage, the fat can be of the usual source and distribution.

What about the mechanics of the system involving the American Diabetes Association Exchange List? This was conceived to relieve the monotony of a dietary regime and is based on classifying all the common foods into six groups: milk products, vegetables, fruits, bread stuffs, meats or pro-teins, and fats. Each food in a group in the amount specified in the tables is approximately equal in caloric equivalence and percentage of carbohydrates to any other food in that group. Thus they may be exchanged one for the other at various meals, thereby alleviating the monotony and permit-ting flexibility and variation in the diet. Basically, this type of dietary regime can be used for any patient who is undergo-ing some modification of his food intake.

There are certain foods marked "dietetic" or "for diabet-ics" that are purportedly lower in sugar and/or carbohydrates than regular foods on the supermarket shelves. However, they can be a trap for the unwary diabetic unless the label is read carefully because they do contain some sugar and they do have a caloric value. They cannot be eaten ad lib or with impunity because of this, and they must be considered in the total calorie count. Patients very often may eat a whole box of dietetic cookies and feel they are not doing anything to increase their weight or to harm themselves, whereas the actual value may be 100 or 200 calories added to the carefully constructed regular diet. It is better to use conventional foods in a proper manner than to use the special foods.

Authorities are not of a unanimous opinion on the use of alcohol by diabetics and one should be guided by his physician. Alcohol does contain calories, and, if imbibed, the amount should be considered in the total daily allowance.

The debate has long raged and is still continuing over just how rigid the dietary management of diabetics should be and just how important it is. Prior to the 1930s dietary mandates were almost universally enforced. Since that time, when the pediatricians forced a break in the extreme strictness of diet, diabetologists have been divided into two camps. One felt that a stringent diet must be imposed, permitting little, if any, deviation from the almost ritualistic preparation and consumption of meals. The other held that diet should be completely free so long as the patient did not have episodes of ketosis or hypoglycemia. The great question that keeps the debate alive and that is essentially unresolved is whether vigorous treatment and control, in which diet is the cornerstone, prevents the complications of diabetes from occurring.

Without trying to settle this basic question, the American Diabetes Association in the September, 1971, issue of its journal, *Diabetes*, stated: "There no longer appears to be a need to restrict disproportionately the intake of carbohydrate in the diet of most diabetic patients."

The statement was the result of deliberation and study by the ADA's Committee on Food and Nutrition.

Is this so radical and new an idea in the dietary management of diabetes? No, it is not. It was proposed very early on and then became lost in the recommendations of physicians who followed. In 1675 Thomas Willis observed that the urine of diabetics was sweet and theorized that the lost sugar should be replaced. He recommended that the diet contain a large carbohydrate element. However, in 1796 John Rollo's work ushered in the era of the low-carbohydrate, high-protein diet that contained plenty of fats. He noted improvement in the diabetics who adhered to this regime. In 1860 Charles H. Pile at the University of Pennsylvania supported Rollo's theory, and the idea of the low-carbohydrate diet became firmly entrenched. Its ultimate expression was in 1914 with the Allen diet, which included starvation until the blood sugar was lowered, then up to 20 grams of carbohydrate in a daily 1,000-calorie allowance.

So from 1796 until 1921 the low-carbohydrate regime was very firmly entrenched. Occasionally, dissident voices cried out for providing higher carbohydrate content to replace the lost sugar. In 1902 Carl Von Noorden proposed a diet high in oats, which contain carbohydrate, and noted that certain of his patients who followed this suggestion had lowered glycosuria (the presence in the urine of abnormal amounts of sugar).

After the discovery of insulin, the voices in favor of increasing the carbohydrate component in diabetic diets grew louder. In 1923 H. Rawle Gegelin of Columbia University felt that when diabetes was due to insulin deficiency, with insulin replacement the patient should be allowed a normal carbohydrate allotment. In his experiments he increased the carbohydrate five times and found that he did not have to increase the insulin dose to keep his patients in reasonable balance. In 1935 Harold Himsworth at the University of London and Walter Kempner, now at Duke University, reported the results of experiments showing the ability of diabetics to tolerate increases in carbohydrates.

However, the fear of high-carbohydrate diets lingered on in influential medical circles, and it took years to diminish. The number of pages devoted to high-carbohydrate diets in the textbooks of the Joslin Clinic were as follows:

1935—6½ pages
1940—3 pages
1946—an italicized section
1952—no mention

So it would seem that the drive toward allowing additional carbohydrates in the diet had been quashed, but once again there were outbreaks. In 1963 Daniel Stone and William E. Konner indicated that they felt additional carbohydrate in patients on insulin would be beneficial. But it was not until 1970, when J. D. Brunzell at the University of Washington substituted carbohydrates for fats while keeping the daily caloric intake the same, that some acceptance was found. His short, eight- to ten-day study showed improved glucose tolerance when the patients were being given either oral hypoglycemic agents or insulin. Why did the study achieve favor? It might appear that it "was an idea whose time had finally come."

Then in 1971 the American Diabetes Association issued its statement on carbohydrate limitation in the diet.

Why is the current idea enjoying acceptance now? After all, it reversed what had always been held as a dominant and sacred theme in the treatment of diabetes—that if the carbohydrate intake were limited, then the management job was being accomplished. The present opinion puts emphasis on a sound ideal, namely the achievement of normal body weight, with more reliance on calories than on a specific amount of carbohydrates. In maintaining low-carbohydrate content with subsequent increase in fats, there may well be a relationship to atherogenesis. Perhaps lower fats and higher carbohydrates may have long-term effects on decreasing blood cholesterol, and thus the buildup of fat in the arteries, which has a deleterious effect, especially in the coronary circulation in the heart.

The ADA pronouncement is not a complete abandonment of dietary principles. The patient must still:

1. Restrict simple sugar to avoid peaks and valleys in blood sugar;
2. Space meals properly for insulin action;
3. Keep to ideal weight by means of caloric limitations.

It has been accepted for years that diabetics can be controlled with the prevailing diet of the area in which they live. In Japan, carbohydrate makes up 64 percent of the food intake, while in India it is 70 percent. A patient's compliance with a dietary order may be improved if it follows the kind of regime familiar to him. In the United States, carbohydrate normally makes up 45 percent of the diet. And note that the ADA says not to restrict the diet "disproportionately." American diabetics may eat the same kinds of foods their families eat; there is no need for special foods to be cooked.

Thus the first step in the treatment of diabetes is the adoption of a diet routine that will bring the patient to his ideal weight. It is certainly possible to treat a great number, if not the majority, of maturity-onset diabetics with diet alone and to establish satisfactory control solely by this means.

Let us say something here about motivation on the part of the patient to control his diabetes by means of diet. There is no doubt that successful adherence to diet is better ensured when the patient is truly stimulated by one means or another to follow the prescription. Dr. Leo P. Krall at the Joslin Clinic is in a unique position on this score—his patients, maturity-onset diabetics, do not cheat on their diets. In fact, as he reported to *Medical World News,* "the biggest difficulty is that they are so anxious to succeed they may not eat enough."

The main reason for this kind of motivation is that the patients are all airline pilots and they would like to keep their satisfying, high-paying jobs. Were they to have to go to insulin or oral hypoglycemic medication to control their diabetes, they would be grounded. The Federal Aviation Agency, which controls the license of an airline pilot, feels that the need for medication to control diabetes is an indicator of the severity of the condition. And severe diabetes could result in hypoglycemia and impairment of judgment.

Dr. Krall is of the opinion that if a pilot's disease can be controlled by diet alone, he should be permitted to fly, since the disease is more potential than active. The required semi-annual pilot physical helps the situation in that it almost guarantees that the disease is detected early.

The diet, low in calories and high in nutrients, is taken on a five-meal-a-day schedule that helps stave off hunger pangs. It starts strictly, to get the patient about 5 percent below normal weight. Those who are overweight go on a severely limited 600-calorie-a-day regime until they reach the desired weight. Thereafter, they go on an 1,800–1,900-calorie maintenance diet that is enough for sustenance but not enough to add weight. His typical 1,540-calorie-a-day prescription would contain 160 grams of carbohydrate, 90 grams of protein, and 60 grams of fat, emphasizing green vegetables, lean meat, a certain amount of fruit, and very little starch.

Dr. Krall's experience with these patients has been refreshing, since the ADA estimates that only 15 percent of patients follow prescribed diets. Through early detection and vigorous dietary measures, his pilot-patients have avoided becoming overt diabetics for as long as ten years.

While the total relationship of obesity to diabetes is not clearly known, perhaps an analogy might help explain the state of present knowledge. A house built with five rooms has a furnace installed that can easily provide the proper amount of heat for the area to be covered. Double the number of rooms, and the furnace's output will not be able to cope with the increased demand. So it is in the pancreas—the Beta cells have the capacity, established at birth, to provide the proper amount of insulin for normal body weight. When fat cells are enlarged and increased in number, the pancreas cannot keep up with the demand, the Beta cells become exhausted, and diabetes ensues. Dr. Jesse Roth at the National Institutes of Health has been working with insulin receptor sites on muscle and fat cells. He has found that when there are a lot of fat cells, there are fewer receptor sites at which the insulin can work. By shrinking the fat cells in reducing the weight, the effectiveness of the receptor sites is enhanced.

It must be recognized that slavish adherence to a rigorous diet has little appeal and will not be universally accepted. Psychological as well as physiological factors play a role in the way reducing diets will be followed—especially by those who most need to lose weight. Therefore, in many patients who are obese or who have difficulty in bringing down their weight, it is sometimes the path of least resistance and greater effectiveness in establishing control to use either insulin or the oral hypoglycemic agents, although this may not be the best physiological means to accomplish it in these people.

As seen in the airline pilots and their approach to diet, motivation plays an important role. If the physician can find in his other patients something to trigger a response to the need for diet, the treatment of maturity-onset diabetics will be much improved.

6

Other Therapy

The keystone in treatment of the diabetic is dietary modification, and in many cases no other measures need be used. However, there will be a number of patients in whom this is impossible, some at the very point of original diagnosis and others whose sugar balance remains poor after some time on a modified diet. In these cases the physician must resort to medication to help maintain the blood sugar at a proper level, which will eliminate the symptoms indicating poor control.

In the present state of medical knowledge, two kinds of administered medication are available, and each should be used in conjunction with a dietary regimen that the physician considers satisfactory and with which the patient can live comfortably. There is insulin, of which there are now a number of types. And there are the various oral hypoglycemic drugs.

Within the broad category of patients who cannot be controlled by diet alone there are those who also cannot be treated with the oral agents. They are either juvenile-onset diabetics or those whose disease showed up later in life but acts similarly to the juvenile type. These people must use insulin or else they will progress rather rapidly into ketoacidosis and diabetic coma.

The discovery of insulin in 1921, of course, changed the complexion of the treatment of diabetes radically because the average diabetic up to that time, even with the most rigorous dietary control, lived only about 6.1 years following the detection of the disease. The use of insulin to control the acute, fulminating ravages of the disease certainly made a remarkable difference in longevity and survival. It also, though, allowed diabetics to live long enough so that they developed some of the complications that may eventually appear after a number of years with the disease.

The discovery of insulin produced an unexpected effect. Since it was available when all other means of control failed, its utilization on a grand scale ushered in an era of nonprogress in both clinical and basic research into the underlying causes and effects of the disease.

It became apparent soon after 1921 that the basic insulin of Banting and Best was short-acting and in need of some kind of modification and improvement so that it would provide a wider range of effectiveness. Thus scientists became involved in research directed at finding the means by which injected insulin could be made to imitate more closely the pancreatic release mechanism in the normal individual—or at least the means to be able to keep a supply of insulin in the bloodstream long enough to react with sugar produced by food intake, thus maintaining a reasonable balance.

By 1936, Hagedorn and his colleagues produced an insulin combined with protamine, a protein material derived from fish sperm which, when injected under the skin, permitted a steady and prolonged absorption of insulin into the bloodstream. The medical world hailed this as the most significant advance in diabetic treatment beyond the discovery of insulin itself. More recently, Lente insulin was developed as a more purified form of the hormone, and this has diminished the number of allergic reactions suffered by some patients in using the other insulins. Of even more recent vintage is a form of insulin called "single-component," which is the purest form yet devised, being 99 percent pure as against the 92 percent purity of Lente, the preparation with the fewest impurities prior to this.

The commercial preparation of insulin is a complicated and lengthy process. It takes several million pounds of raw pancreases from animals each year to provide the supply of insulin that finally reaches patients. The processors get one pound of zinc-insulin crystals from 10,000 pounds of beef and pork pancreases. These are frozen immediately after slaughter to prevent destruction of insulin by pancreatic enzymes and then are ground up into 100- to 150-pound batches. Then comes treatment with acid alcohol, which extracts the insulin and also suppresses any further activity of the other enzymes. The gland residue is treated with alkali to precipitate out the impurities. The extract is made acid again and the alcohol is removed. The substance is warmed to remove fat, which rises to the top, permitting the lower layers to be filtered, taking out insoluble impurities. The concentrated extract is treated with salt, the insulin precipitates, and the process is repeated until it is of the desired purity, then crystallized, washed, and dried.

What is a unit of insulin? It is a reference standard for potency, originally based on the amount of the preparation required to bring down the blood sugar of a normal rabbit, 2 kilograms (4.4 pounds) in weight, after 24-hour fasting, from 120 mg% to 45 mg% in a five-hour period. However, with improved manufacturing techniques it became possible to obtain a potent, reproducible extract, and this became a standard against which all batches were tested. Now, instead of measuring the unit by the physiological reaction of the rabbit, it is based on an absolute weight of insulin prepared from a recrystallized composite sample.

Depending on the patient's life-style and severity of disease, the physician will prescribe a specific type of insulin or combination of insulins in order to achieve and maintain a proper metabolic balance. Also prescribed will be the dosage necessary to achieve the desired effect. There are three main categories of insulin in present use—short-acting, intermediate in effect, and long-lasting. In the first group is the unmodified regular and Semilente; in the second is Lente, NPH, and globin; while in the third is PZI (protamine zinc) and Ultralente. All of these come in different strengths—U-40, U-80, and U-100. The U-40 contains 40 units of insulin in one milliliter, and the U-80 provides 80 units per milliliter. The U-100, with 100 units per milliliter, is comparatively new and offers a number of advantages. It will reduce the possibility of error since it is to be used only with a U-100 syringe and no arithmetical calculation of dosage need be made; it requires less quantity to achieve the same effect the lower-strength insulins provide; and it will cut down on the cost of production. Most hospitals have welcomed the U-100 insulin, and it will probably be accepted universally as the strength to be prescribed.

Since the production of insulin relies directly on the supply of animal pancreases, attempts have been made to produce it synthetically. Working completely independently of each other, but seemingly parallel in thought, Helmut Zahn of West Germany, P. G. Katsoyannis at the University of Pittsburgh, and a group of Chinese researchers in Shanghai about ten years ago announced chemical synthesis almost at the same time. However, so far it is not possible to prepare synthetic insulin in sufficient quantity to make it available for clinical use. It is an extremely complex process, requiring 234 separate and distinct chemical reactions.

When the diabetic uses insulin he cannot further control its action. Once having injected the prescribed dose, he is literally stuck with it and is then committed to taking in the right amount of food to balance the insulin already injected. If he does not do so, he runs the risk of undergoing an insulin reaction or insulin shock. The normal individual doesn't need to think about this because his pancreas will produce the proper amount of insulin in response to the glucose load presented to it. Even with the most meticulous control of food intake and the judicious, measured use of insulin of various types, it is almost impossible to approximate the action of the normal pancreas. Work is being done on this problem and it is possible that new knowledge will be able to help solve it in the future. The use of a number of types of insulin taken at different times, short-acting and long-acting, is sometimes referred to as "insulin calisthenics" and is a vigorous attempt to mimic the activity of the normal pancreas.

A summary of the kinds of insulin now available, their action times and time at which an insulin reaction or shock is most likely to take place, follows. The table has been made up with the assumption that the dosage of insulin will be taken shortly before breakfast.

There are authorities in diabetes, among them Dr. George F. Cahill, Jr., professor of medicine at the Harvard Medical School and director of the Joslin Research Laboratory, who recommend strongly that juvenile-onset diabetics take three insulin injections a day: regular insulin before breakfast and lunch, and a mixture of regular and Lente or NPH insulin before dinner to carry the patient through the night. While this might help to keep the blood glucose as nearly normal as possible, most people would find it a very trying routine and some would deem it impossible. Thus the physician prescribes a combination of insulins, and the times for injection, that will help the patient as well as conforming to the lifestyle. The most important principle in treatment by means of insulin is that each patient requires individual management.

While it may be considered advisable to hospitalize some

Insulin Preparations and Their Action

| Type | Action (by hour) | | | Insulin Reaction Most Likely to Occur |
	Start	Strongest Activity	Length of Action	
I. Quick-acting				
Regular	½	2–4	6–8	Late morning
Semilente	1	6–10	12–16	Late morning
II. Intermediate				
Globin	2–4	6–12	12–20	Late afternoon
Lente	2–4	8–12	28–32	Late afternoon
NPH	2–4	8–12	18–30	Late afternoon
III. Extended-duration				
Protamine zinc	3–6	14–20	24–36	Night and very early morning
Ultralente	9	16–24	up to 48	Night and very early morning

newly diagnosed diabetics for special evaluation and to start therapy, most of the time all the procedures can be performed in the physician's office. In addition to the discussions with the patient—explanation of the condition and the details of the therapy—the family must also be educated concerning the disease and the treatment. The close relatives, especially those with whom the patient lives, have to understand the correlation among diet, exercise, and insulin requirements under various conditions. They should also be made aware of the signs of insulin shock, as well as ketoacidosis, and what must be done quickly to aid the patient.

The diabetic should recognize that regular exercise is important in the total management of his condition, not only because of the consequent heightened sensitivity of the body cells to insulin action but also because it is beneficial to the entire cardiovascular system. It is possible to lower the blood sugar to an extent by exercise alone, but beyond that exercise will, if a person is in good physical condition because of regular participation in sports or similar activity, help circulation, improve muscle tone, and generally make for feeling of well being. The diabetic who takes part in regular exercise must evaluate his insulin requirements so that the reduction of blood sugar through activity will not add too much to the decrease due to the insulin, resulting in a hypoglycemic state and insulin shock. This can be done through experiment and observation and should not be considered such a worrisome matter that the exercise is foresworn. There are some great athletes who are diabetics, and their means of solving the problem is to plan ahead so they do not take more insulin than necessary before a game or match. William Talbert, the tennis player, and Bobby Clarke, the star hockey player with the Philadelphia Flyers, are two excellent examples of coping with the diabetic state while still remaining at the top of their respective classes in sports.

Regular exercise tends to reduce the dosage requirement for insulin, so once the level of activity is correlated with the need for insulin, a balance can easily be achieved. What needs to be avoided is a sudden, unplanned increase in effort that might then result in an insulin reaction. To prevent this, the diabetic should always carry with him some hard candy or a packet of sugar, which can then be taken at the first sign of an insulin reaction.

Essential in a treatment plan for diabetics is the prevention of infection of the lower limbs and the feet. For the reason that diabetics handle infection rather poorly, prevention is certainly better than treatment. In the lower limbs, because of possible diminution in sensation due to nerve damage and because of changes caused by decreased circulation, infections may not be noticed at their start. The sensation of pain may be dulled, and once infections occur they may not heal properly because of poor blood supply. In addition to these obvious things, there seems to be some special problem, the cause as yet undetermined, that diabetics face in their basic response to infection. It may well be that the high blood sugar in diabetics provides a good biological medium for bacterial growth, but even well-controlled diabetics may also have a greater tendency toward infection.

Cognizant of this, the physician will examine the feet of his diabetic patient carefully at each office visit. He will check for signs of diminished circulation; decreased sensation; any indications of poorly fitted shoes such as redness, blisters, or irritated areas; and specific symptoms that may portend future problems. The physician will prescribe certain procedures for the patient to follow, and these should be scrupulously performed.

The retina of the eye not only provides information concerning intrinsic eye damage because of diabetes but is also an indicator of the general health of the entire cardiovascular system. Each examination of the eyes includes a searching inspection of the retina and its network of blood vessels, which may express, by early warning signs, evidence of forthcoming problems in the eye itself as well as in the arteries and veins in other parts of the body. Usually the first thing the physician sees is small red dots, which are tiny aneurysms in the blood vessels. Further on in the progress of the disease may come detached retinas and vision problems.

Up to a few years ago the physician could not help the diabetic who began to show the proliferating abnormal blood vessels in the retina. However, the disease itself can now be slowed down through the use of the laser beam. Aimed at the back of the eye in extremely precise fashion, this thin beam of light goes through the lens of the eye, focusing on the offending blood vessel. It seals the leak, and the process is repeated as many times as there are spots that need to be closed. This operation causes no pain and is most effective when the vessel problems are in their early stages.

Probably one of the most exciting developments in the treatment of diabetes, after insulin and its modifications for long-lasting effect, was the arrival on the scene of the oral antidiabetic agents. Since insulin is a protein, it is ineffective when swallowed because the digestive enzymes in the stomach destroy it before it can be absorbed into the bloodstream. Thus the only means of administering insulin is by injection into the body by hypodermic needle.

In 1948 two French medical scientists, R. Jonbon and A. L. Loubatiéres, in the course of studying the effects of antibiotics noticed that some of their experimental mice developed symptoms similar to hypoglycemia. In following this up, they observed that those mice who were treated with certain sulfa compounds did show low blood sugars. The scientists then became deeply involved with the whole question of oral hypoglycemic agents.

What resulted from this original research and then further work by many people was the discovery of two large categories of drugs which, when taken orally, reduced the blood sugars in diabetics. These classifications are: the sulfonylureas which are marketed as Orinase, Tolinase, Diabinese, and Dymelor; and the biguanides, which are DBI and Meltrol. These oral agents will not be effective in diabetics who have an absolute deficiency of insulin. Remember that the juvenile-onset diabetic has been shown through radioimmunoassay tests to be utterly devoid of internally produced insulin, while the maturity-onset patient usually secretes some of the hormone. In the latter the insulin may not be effective because of problems in the transport or absorption processes, but the oral agents will work where there is some of the hormone present.

The sulfonylureas' chief activity seems to be to stimulate the pancreas to secrete additional insulin in those diabetics whose output is inadequate. This has been noted in a number of experimental animals where the primary action of these compounds was in the pancreas. There is some question, however, whether these agents may increase the breakdown of pro-insulin to insulin or perform at the cellular level to sensitize the cell to the action of insulin, or perhaps they may act in some way in the liver. It may be that the sulfonylureas act at any of these points, but the evidence is not yet clearly at hand concerning the mode of action.

The biguanides were initially thought to perform by making insulin more effective at the cellular level. More recent research has shown that a major role is in inhibiting the absorption of glucose in the intestine, therefore reducing the amount that gets into the blood.

In 1960 a major study was started, called the University Group Diabetes Program, which sought to evaluate the role of diet alone, insulin, and an oral agent, Orinase (Tolbutamide), in the treatment of diabetes. The study was originally conceived to be evaluative in the comparative treatment of diabetes by these means and was undertaken by twelve centers in the United States and Puerto Rico, involving about 800 diabetics. The patients were divided into four equal groups, one to be treated by diet alone, the second to be given Orinase on a fixed-dose schedule, the third on a fixed dose of insulin, and the fourth on a variable amount of insulin depending on blood sugar values.

The benefits of Orinase that had been cited prior to the study and after it was first accepted were certainly its convenience, its ability to treat diabetics who could not be controlled by diet alone, and its easy use by elderly patients who could not adhere to diet and yet were unable to take insulin because of poor eyesight, fear of the injection, or arthritis of the hands that made using the syringe difficult.

After the study was under way and the scientists had begun to analyze the data, one of the unexpected results that came to light, in 1969, was that patients in the study who were taking Orinase had a greater number of deaths from heart attacks than did any of the other groups—twice as many, as a matter of fact. Similar experiences were observed in a corollary portion of the study dealing with DBI. This led to tremendous controversy among physicians and has divided the field of diabetologists into two large camps. There were those who felt that the accumulated data were not proof positive for one reason or another, and that Orinase was a valuable, useful, and safe drug. There were those who were convinced that on the basis of this definitive statistical increase in mortality from heart attacks, Orinase should no longer be used. The argument is still raging in the medical literature and at medical meetings, with no resolution although there are compelling arguments on both sides. Nevertheless, in the face of the evidence concerning the death rate from heart attacks, after eight years the study was discontinued.

One of the major criticisms of the UGDP study report revolved around its biostatistical aspects and the charges by opponents that the validity of these was open to serious question.

In response to these charges and to determine the accuracy of the findings, the National Institutes of Health commissioned the prestigious Biometric Society to appoint a panel of distinguished biostatisticians who would assess the studies in detail. They reported their findings in February, 1975, and the judgment was that the oral antidiabetic pills were probably capable of causing premature death from heart disease.

In an editorial on February 10, 1975, in the *Journal of the American Medical Association,* Dr. Thomas C. Chalmers, president of the Mount Sinai Medical Center in New York City, cited the two retrospective studies of variously treated diabetics at the Joslin Clinic in Boston and the Mayo Clinic in Rochester, Minnesota. The one at the Joslin Clinic included 2,167 patients and that at the Mayo Clinic was of 1,470. Wrote Dr. Chalmers:

> . . . Both studies included newly diagnosed cases of diabetes in patients over 40 years old who were treated with only one form of therapy for more than 90 per cent of the time. After correcting for risk factors, both studies revealed increased death rates among patients treated with oral hypoglycemics for more than three years in the Mayo series and more than five years in the Joslin series. . . .

Dr. Chalmers also stated that after the two clinics stopped using the oral agents they found that in many patients there was little or no change in the blood glucose values, indicating, he said, that there was no need for the drugs in the first place. Many of the patients could be controlled by diet alone, some just with mild restriction. Others required rigid dietary management and/or insulin to keep them in balance.

Even though Dr. Chalmers is held in high esteem in the biomedical community, his editorial was not universally accepted as the last word in the controversy. So the argument still goes on.

It is important to note, in discussing this subject fully, that the United States Food and Drug Administration has recommended that the treatment of diabetes should be first diet, then insulin, and, as a last resort in patients who cannot use insulin, the oral antidiabetic agents. Let us emphasize also that the objective of therapy, by whatever means chosen, is to establish as nearly as good a physiological situation concerning blood sugar balance in the diabetic as exists in the nondiabetic.

The ultimate decision concerning the mode of therapy to be followed must rest with the individual physician, who should inform the patient of the controversy evoked by the UGDP study as part of the decision-making process. He must take a course that he considers best for his patient, weighing all of the factors known to him.

Ideal control is seldom realized, so compromises must be made. Most physicians consider a patient to be in satisfactory control if the following criteria are met:

1. The patient feels well and has no symptoms of hypoglycemia or hyperglycemia. His clinical status is what would be considered normal and asymptomatic.

2. The patient's weight is stable and at a level consistent with accepted standards.

3. The results of urine analysis tests should usually run

between "negative" and "1 +" sugar on most of the tests performed. Traces are completely acceptable, but heavy glycosuria at times is not a sign of uncontrol.

4. While blood sugars are difficult to interpret, most physicians feel that fasting blood sugars under 150 mg% and two-hour postprandial sugars under 200 mg% are felt to be compatible with good control. There are great variations possible in this, so the individual physician must determine whether his patient is in good control with these values, or as an alternate must set other values for the patient to maintain.

5. The lipid metabolism should be within normal limits, as indicated by the demonstration of normal cholesterol and triglycerides in the blood.

6. The patient should function well enough to live a useful, normal, and happy life, with a respect for his illness but not a terror of it, so that the quality of his life as well as the quantity is something desirable.

The maintenance of good control is no simple matter and indeed may even be impossible under present-day circumstances. A recent study by George Molnar of the Mayo Clinic brought out some interesting points. In a group of diabetics who were thought to be well controlled in the sense discussed above, he measured glucose levels at intervals of one to two hours over a twenty-four-hour period. When the results were analyzed, in the course of a day during which they were working, exercising, eating, etc., it was found that 90 percent of the time their blood sugars were either above or below the acceptable norms. So even in those patients in whom there is as good control as can be achieved with insulin administration once or twice a day, the situation is still poor when compared with the normal activity of the pancreas. However, even though the patient may not be in really good control under the best treatment procedure, and does not approximate a normal situation, he and his physician should continue to strive for better management because even an approach to normalcy will help in the long run of the disease.

The basic reason for the emphasis on controlling the blood sugar content is that there is strong feeling, but not unanimity, that the closer he approaches normal blood sugar control, the less likely it will be that he would develop the complications related to diabetes. And yet control may not be the whole story, since studies by Dr. David Rimoin, chief of the division of medical genetics at Harbor General Hospital, Torrance, California, seem to indicate a possibility that the blood sugar level and vascular changes may not be related but may have different genetic bases. This would account for the fact that one diabetic with long-term high blood sugar will not fall heir to the diabetic complications while another will come down with all the sequelae. In the same vein, the Pima Indians of Arizona suffer a very high rate of diabetes but have a low rate of vascular, eye, or kidney complications. On the other hand, among the Amish people of Pennsylvania the diabetes is followed by all the complications that can beset a diabetic after a number of years with the disease.

Supporting good control is the Joslin Clinic experience described earlier in which well-controlled diabetics showed relatively few complications over a long period of time.

Albert Winegrad, professor of medicine at the University of Pennsylvania, and his associates have shown that, in the presence of high blood sugar, large amounts of a substance known as sorbitol is produced in certain tissues. Sorbitol has the ability to distort the lens of the eye and also affects the lining of certain arteries. It is believed that certain complications of diabetes are directly related to the sorbitol pathway.

The course of diabetes in experimental animals in which the pancreatic islet cells have been destroyed also tends to support the thesis that diabetic complications are secondary to the blood glucose levels. In the recent work of Dr. J. M. B.

Bloodworth, professor of pathology at the University of Wisconsin Medical School, where he took two groups of diabetic dogs, treated one group vigorously to keep blood sugars within acceptable bounds, and treated the other group just enough to keep them from dying, evidence is disclosed that vigorous control of the glucose levels can avert the development of complications. After five years of the experiment, the dogs were sacrificed and postmortem examination found few vascular lesions in the controlled dogs but many in the uncontrolled group.

The physician not only treats the patient, he also treats the abnormal biochemistry present in diabetes. Thus an abnormal finding cannot be ignored just because the patient feels well.

Advocating good treatment that leads to optimum control might well be compared to coming out for motherhood and against sin. The ultimate aim of therapy, however it is carried out, is the maintenance of a happy, functioning patient who can live the kind of life he enjoys without having it cut short by complications.

7

Research

Research! A magic word, one to conjure with, a term that piques the imagination. Research! Its connotation evokes images of dedicated scientists in pristine white endlessly peering into bubbling test tubes or manipulating complicated gadgetry, shouting "Eureka" from time to time or stating with magnificently weary understatement, "Now I think we've got it," then going out to announce yet another medical mystery fathomed. Impressed by medical research and the mystique surrounding it, prominent philanthropists and great foundations have made munificent grants of funds. Caught up in the demand of the public for cures and by its fear of disease, the Congress of the United States has appropriated billions of dollars over the years to establish and support the National Institutes of Health, our country's most prestigious biomedical research organization.

All research, whatever the motivation, whether to add to knowledge generally or to solve a particular problem specifically, starts essentially with curiosity. The inquiring mind begins with the objective of gaining information about something that is obscure or to add to understanding of an area that is not well known.

Sometimes the result is accidental—before the apple fell on Isaac Newton's head he probably had not even thought of defining and phrasing the Law of Gravity.

Similarly, the discovery of one of the most powerful antibiotic drugs, penicillin, came about through accident. Sir Alexander Fleming, in studying factors inhibiting the growth of organisms, had cultures of staphylococci, a kind of bacteria, growing in his laboratory at St. Mary's Hospital in London. It was the summer of 1929, and the weather was cool and damp, when a mold borne up the stairs by the wind alighted on the culture plate. This is a common mishap in a bacteriological laboratory, and usually the contaminated plate is washed by a lab assistant and the contents discarded. On this particular day, however, Dr. Fleming himself inspected his plates and found that the colonies of staphylococci around the intruding mold had begun to disappear. He then determined that the mold was of the genus *Penicillium* and that it acted on some bacterial organisms but had no effect on others. After further tests, he predicted that someday it would be used as an effective and powerful therapeutic agent. So it was, after a number of years of refinement, improvement, and processing. But the original discovery was truly an accident—a serendipitous one, to be sure, but completely unforeseen nevertheless.

Dr. Albert Einstein studied mathematics and its application to physical principles in matter. His theory of relativity and the properties of matter resulted in the now famous formula $E = mc^2$, which elucidated a function of energy but also provided the basic knowledge for nuclear fission. The first application was in the atomic bomb, but the same principle is being applied in nuclear power plants for ships and submarines as well as in the generation of electrical power for cities.

Obviously, not all research accomplishes its mission through accident. Many projects have been started with a defined goal and have proceeded down the road to fruition. One example is the development of the poliomyelitis vaccine, which first depended on the isolation and identification of the disease-causing virus. When this was done after years of painstaking effort on the part of Dr. John Enders and his virology group at Harvard University, the door was opened for Dr. Jonas Salk to make the killed-virus vaccine first used for prevention and then for Dr. Albert Sabin to take the process one step further and perfect the live but weakened virus vaccine that has been used all over the world. The entire project, from start to finish, was aimed toward the goal of immunization. It moved unswervingly on its way until the vaccine was in general use, effectively wiping out poliomyelitis as a menace to health.

Research in any field, whether in medicine or in the manufacture of manmade fibers for clothing, takes two forms— basic and applied (sometimes called targeted). Basic research is performed primarily to increase or intensify knowledge and is usually a laborious, less exciting, and less thrilling occupation than applied research. Basic research is involved with determining mechanisms and processes, causes and modes of action. Applied research, on the other hand, is occupied with solving specific problems in the best way possible. In the field of genetics, for example, basic research works with the description, identification, and function of DNA (deoxyribonucleic acid), called familiarly "the building blocks of life," and RNA (ribonucleic acid), which has another function in the cell. Applied research in genetics would concern itself with genetic engineering, genetic counseling, and determining the mode of inheritance of various characteristics.

Among the metabolic disorders plaguing the human race, diabetes is now the one probably most intensively studied.

Research has taken the form of concentrated studies designed to gain an improved understanding of the underlying causes of the disease. While two decades ago there were only a few centers devoted to studying diabetes, there is now almost worldwide participation, with centers in New York, Boston, Geneva, and South Africa leading the way. One result of the increased interest and expanded work has been the exponential increase in the number of research papers presented at meetings of the American Diabetes Association and the International Diabetes Federation, attesting to the additional scientists and centers working on the problems.

Since the immediate objective in diabetes appears to be the achievement of good management so that the patient can live a reasonably normal life, much of the investigation is in the form of applied research aimed at improved control of the blood sugar—keeping it within narrow and normal limits. Much time, effort, and financial support are being devoted to this, with a certain amount of progress noted. However, it is almost axiomatic in medicine that the best solution is most often the least expensive and least complicated. In poliomyelitis, for instance, alleviation of the damage done by the disease—the use of the iron lung and other respirators, constant application of hot packs, development of braces and crutches to deal with the paralytic limbs—was expensive and not truly a satisfactory way of dealing with polio. The same thing is true in coronary artery disease, which now is treated fairly often by means of the coronary artery bypass operation, an open-heart procedure that is expensive and a rather drastic method of providing relief. How much better it would be were there a simple and easy means of preventing the blockage of the coronary circulation. The accomplishments of applied research in polio, it is readily seen, pale into insignificance against the accomplishment of the vaccine that, for a few pennies per dose, in effect eliminated the disease. True, the development costs were great, but not when measured against the cost of treatment and rehabilitation of the victims.

So it would be with diabetes, too. Even if methods for ideally regulating the blood sugar were to be perfected tomorrow, how much better and how much more economical of time, money, and suffering it would be were there a true comprehension of the basic cause of diabetes and a means discovered of preventing its occurrence.

This ultimate discovery will come only from the knowledge gained in basic research, so no matter what promise applied research holds out for the immediate relief of the clinical manifestations of diabetes, basic research must not be diminished; it must even be increased in magnitude and scope.

Senator Edward M. Kennedy, in a report submitted to accompany the proposed National Diabetes Research and Education Act placed before the Senate in 1973, stated:

> . . . The present state of knowledge of the vascular complications of diabetes can only be described as very inadequate. Involvement of the larger vessels takes the form of cerebral, coronary and peripheral arteriosclerosis leading to strokes, heart attacks and gangrene. In diabetics these changes occur at a much earlier age and in more severe degree than in nondiabetics. Fully as important as such disease of the larger vessels is disease of the small vessels, known as microangiopathy, which takes the vision and then the life of many young diabetics. This small vessel disease is specifically related to diabetes and eventually occurs in almost all of the tissues of the body of all diabetics if they live long enough. It manifests itself most destructively in the eyes and in the kidneys.
>
> Much remains to be done. Not enough is known about diabetic vascular disease to apply scientific knowledge to its prevention and treatment. Acquisition of knowledge of biological phenomena usually goes through three phases: first, discovery or recognition; second, description, and finally, precise definitions of the mechanisms involved. In

the case of diabetic vascular complications, medical science has toiled through the phases of recognition and description but has only made a start on the difficult research task of defining the biological mechanisms by which these changes in the blood vessel walls come about. Research in this area, as well as in many other areas of diabetes, must be encouraged and supported if we are ever to have effective preventive measures and treatment.

Although it is important to detect diabetes early and educate both the physician and the patient for optimal care, it is only as a consequence of expanded research in diabetes and related diseases that we can hope to avoid the ever-increasing economic and emotional toll which the diabetic and the Nation are bearing.

. . . Modern diabetes research is focused upon finding the cause of the disease. . . . Much of this research is devoted to studies on insulin, how it is produced and released, and how it does its vital work. Scientists believe that this and related fundamental research is the key to understanding diabetes and to improving its treatment.

Other studies have been concerned with the question as to whether the small blood vessel disease characteristic of diabetes is an independent primary cause or an effect of long-term diabetes, and the possible role played by human growth hormones. In addition, there are a number of ongoing investigations of new approaches with a therapeutic potential, such as implantation of insulin-producing pancreatic Beta cells and various studies designed to understand better, and perhaps to forestall, developments of the long-term complications of the disease . . .

The National Diabetes Research and Education Act was passed by Congress and has provided research and education financial support, as well as establishing the National Task Force on Diabetes. The original bill was to allocate funds that would eventually rise to the level of about $30 million per year by the fiscal year 1977. The task force, of fifteen members, has been appointed and is carrying out its assigned duty, which in abbreviated form is, as specified in the act, to:

> formulate a long-range plan to combat diabetes with specific recommendations concerning the utilization and organization of national resources for that purpose after conducting a comprehensive study and survey investigating the magnitude of diabetes mellitus, its epidemiology, its economic and social consequences, and an evaluation of available scientific information and the national resources capable of dealing with the problem. . . .

It is now well accepted that there are truly two types of diabetes mellitus. One is the juvenile-onset disease in which the appearance of symptoms is sudden, intense, and fulminating, giving rise to a ferocious manifestation of the disease within a very short period of time. The other is the milder, slower-developing and less intense form—maturity-onset diabetes mellitus. It is also understood now that in the former either no insulin whatsoever is produced by the great majority of patients or it is of no consequence, but in the latter the hormone is secreted in some quantity.

In considering the juvenile-onset form, scientists have given some credence to the possibility that a causative agent might be viral in nature. One group of researchers, at the State University of New York at Buffalo, studied the incidence in New York's Erie County for the twenty-year period starting in 1947 and then compared this with the occurrence of mumps in the country as a whole. They found that there were peaks and valleys in the amount of mumps and these corresponded to peaks and valleys in a graph of diabetes cases four years later. Since mumps is a "slow" virus that can remain in the pancreas for up to four years, the effect on diabetes is not obvious until several years after exposure. The investigators also correlated their data to the incidence of diabetes among teen-aged boys between 1950 and 1960. This, they felt, was due to the popular notion of exposing adolescent boys to mumps before puberty to prevent the risk of sterility, which is believed to occur if the disease is contracted after puberty. One of the suggestions made by the research group was that medical science should perfect and use a killed-virus vaccine rather than one that contained the live organism. The latter gives the patient a little bit of mumps and then confers immunity, but the researchers felt that if there were truly a link between mumps and diabetes, then even a little bit of mumps was too much. Dr. Harry Sultz of the State University at Buffalo hypothesized in a report to the American Public Health Association in 1975 that when the mumps virus lodges in the pancreas it sets up a reaction in which the insulin-producing cells are slowly damaged, thereby eventually causing juvenile-onset diabetes.

Another study, of diabetes in guinea pigs, which seems to indicate that an infectious process is involved, is being conducted by Dr. Bryce L. Munger at the Pennsylvania State University. He has found, in one of his experiments, that when healthy guinea pigs were placed in a cage with one diabetic guinea pig, half become frankly diabetic within two to six weeks. Dr. Munger reported that these acutely ill animals have elevated blood sugar levels with sugar in the urine, show positive glucose tolerance tests, and have high blood cholesterol levels. Efforts to identify the infectious agent or the mode of transmission so far have not been successful.

The hypothesis concerning a possible infectious cause is given weight by evidence that "epidemic" occurrences of diabetes are reported from time to time in various areas. In addition, one study conducted in England has found that 85 percent of juvenile-onset diabetes mellitus is preceded by an infection. The relationship of diabetes to Coxsackie Virus infections is being extensively studied in the United States.

An area of basic research being vigorously pursued by a number of scientists is the mechanism by which insulin is transported from its source in the Beta cell to the blood-stream. It is known that the maturity-onset diabetic does have insulin-producing capability, but that something goes awry either in the transport system or in the insulin's action at the cell-membrane level, where it normally acts. Defects at these so-called receptor sites have been shown to produce diabetes in experimental models. Dr. Albert Renold and his group in Geneva, Switzerland, have demonstrated in their intensive studies that there is a marked difference between the normal person and the diabetic in the pancreatic insulin production and delivery mechanism. While the ultimate value of these data is not yet clear, they may be basic to the cause of certain types of diabetes. The scientists in Geneva have used freeze-dried electron microscopy to confirm that the secretion of insulin involves the fusion of secretion granules within the Beta cell membrane, but the mechanism of regulation is not yet known. The goal of another research project is to take the Beta cell apart and determine how it regulates insulin secretion in its membrane.

The entire question of the relationship of a group of hormones produced in the brain, and the study of areas in the brain that in part regulate the blood sugar levels, are also under intensive investigation. These studies are laborious, painstaking, and not very glamorous, and imminent translation into immediate benefit to the diabetic population is very remote. But work such as this may eventually provide the basic answer to the riddle of diabetes.

One of the most exciting concepts that has come to the fore in recent years and that has achieved a high degree of acceptance is contradictory of the long-established dogma that diabetes is caused solely by a lack of insulin. Instead, diabetes is now being studied as a multihormonal disturbance in that another hormone, called glucagon and secreted by the Alpha cells of the pancreas, plays a vital role in the etiology of diabetes. It works by causing a substance called glycogen to break down and produce glucose.

Metabolically, insulin and glucagon are opponents. Insulin lowers blood sugar, glucagon causes it to rise.

Leading the way in the basic research into the causal mechanisms that have produced the formulation of the multi-hormone "double trouble" theory is Dr. Roger H. Unger of the University of Texas Southwestern Medical School. After he had studied the glucagon-insulin relationship for more than twenty years, his recent findings strongly support the thesis that the blood sugar balance is controlled by interaction between glucagon and insulin. He has demonstrated that diabetes results not only from an insufficiency of insulin but also because glucagon in the diabetic is produced in excessive amounts. This stimulates the production of more glucose than the insulin can control, thus intensifying the problem of maintaining a good blood sugar balance. When the normal person eats carbohydrate foods, the glucagon production immediately decreases markedly, according to Dr. Unger's findings, but not in diabetics. Through some fault in the internal structure, there is continued secretion of glucagon, which raises the blood sugar level.

The work with glucagon more than suggests a path for future research into means of suppressing excessive glucagon secretion so that administered insulin can be more effective in maintaining the blood sugar at an optimum level. Dr. Unger has stated that this is now a major goal of many researchers. He has also said that until 1974 nobody could claim that suppression of glucagon would ameliorate diabetes, but that this can now be said unequivocally. It has been shown that suppression does result in a remarkable drop in the blood sugar.

During their research, Dr. Unger and his associates removed the pancreases of experimental animals and found that glucagon was still present in the blood. Considering this impossible because they had proceeded on the premise that glucagon was made only in the Alpha cells of the pancreas, they looked further. They found that there were cells similar to the Alphas located at the top of the stomach and in the upper half of the small intestine, merrily producing glucagon at a great rate! When these were removed, the injected insulin became effective once more and the diabetes was brought under control. This reaffirmed the hypothesis that glucagon activity is a very important factor in the pathology of diabetes.

Dr. Unger has expressed optimism about the eventual discovery of an effective glucagon suppressor. He has also said that once this is done and a good blood sugar balance achieved on a continuing basis, then it can be determined whether the complications of diabetes will be helped by improved treatment.

His optimism was well founded, it appears, because in a remarkably fortuitous development in research, a hormone that will suppress the action of glucagon has been identified and isolated. The hormone is known as somatostatin and is found throughout the brain, but particularly in the hypothalamus.

Somatostatin was isolated at the Salk Institute in La Jolla, California, by a team of scientists headed by Dr. Roger Guillemin and Dr. Paul Barzeau during the progress of a long-standing program that was studying the factors causing the pituitary gland to release specific hormones. The releasing factors are produced in the hypothalamic portion of the base of the brain. The group isolated two factors, one causing release of the hormone that affects the gonads (sex glands), and one that controls the thyroid gland. They then began searching for the factor that released somatotrophin, the growth hormone. Instead, they found an inhibitor of the growth hormone and named it somatostatin.

While its obvious use lay in the treatment of conditions such as acromegalic gigantism, a growth aberration, it was found in experiments at the University of Washington in Seattle that somatostatin reduced the blood sugar levels in baboons. Later investigations at the University of California in San Francisco have shown that somatostatin, when given simultaneously with insulin in human diabetics, brings blood sugar levels down markedly lower than those achieved by insulin alone.

It appears that somatostatin has come along at just the right time, its effect coinciding with the discoveries concerning glucagon activity and influence in diabetes. It suppresses both glucagon and insulin, but since the juvenile-type diabetic secretes little or no insulin, the main effect of the somatostatin is on the glucagon. It does not affect insulin that is circulating in the blood. Its influence on the blood sugar level is therefore nothing short of dramatic.

At present the work with somatostatin being done at the University of California by Dr. John D. Gerich of the metabolic research unit is purely experimental. One of the problems in its clinical use is the short duration of its activity in the body. The Salk Institute people are working on a variant that will be longer-lasting and permit a dosage rate of twice a day. Another goal of the research is to modify the hormone molecule so that it does not also inhibit insulin secretion. This would clear the way for use in those diabetics who do secrete some insulin.

Dr. Gerich has said that he anticipates the day, perhaps by 1980, when insulin and somatostatin will be combined into one dose as the treatment of choice for diabetics. This will be, perhaps, most important in diabetes management, but Dr. Gerich has also pointed out publicly that it still does not solve the fundamental conundrum in diabetes. This, of course, is wherein lies the cause of the defective Alpha and Beta cells when the former provide an uncontrolled secretion of glucagon and the latter furnish an inadequate supply of insulin.

The most obvious clinical manifestation of diabetes, the one whose action produces the disease symptoms, is the instability of the blood sugar. Since it seems beneficial to try to keep the sugar as close to normal levels as possible most of the time, and because insulin as presently utilized does this rather imperfectly, researchers have turned their efforts toward supplying the diabetic with a flow of insulin that more nearly approaches the normal.

There are four measures available to simulate normal insulin delivery in the diabetic that are being studied with great interest. First, whole pancreas transplants; second, transplants of the Beta cells; third, stimulation and possible regeneration of weak or exhausted Beta cells; and fourth, an artificial pancreas.

Whole pancreas transplants were probably first considered because of the results of heart transplants, which demonstrated that this technique, though difficult, was feasible and certainly could be attempted. From 1966 to 1975, 36 cases had been performed worldwide, with the longest survival being slightly over one year. Most of these were transplants of the pancreas and kidney in patients with diabetic renal disease.

Many problems cropped up in the pancreatic transplants. First was that the survival time was much too short to determine if the diabetic vascular deterioration was reversed by providing truly normal insulin activity. Second was the rejection phenomenon, which is common to all transplants but which seems to be especially accelerated in pancreas and kidney transplants. Third was the technical difficulty in doing the procedure because part of the gastrointestinal tract, the duodenum, also had to be transplanted, since the pancreas tended to leak at its cut surfaces and to form abscesses. Thus many intraabdominal problems developed after surgery. Fourth was that the use of immunosuppressive drugs such as cortisone to overcome organ rejection makes the diabetic state worse, tending to counteract in a way some of the hoped-for benefits derived from this difficult procedure. Fifth, because diabetics are also extremely sensitive to infection, and the use of immunosuppressive medication will make all people more susceptible, another problem had to be faced. Finally, the financial considerations involved for only one case made this an unfeasible and unrealistic manner of treating diabetes. Added to this is the important problem of donor availability, which has hardly been solved in other organ transplant situations.

So this treatment has been almost completely abandoned by most centers except, perhaps, in very rare instances. It is much too cumbersome, too expensive, too impractical; and in the last analysis the survival rate was very poor. Pancreatic transplantation enjoyed a brief popularity, did not become a means that could be applied as a solution to the diabetic problem, but did prove that the pancreas could be transplanted. It might be likened to crossing Niagara Falls on a tightrope—it can be done, but it is not the easiest or best way to get across.

While the attempts were made to transplant the entire pancreas, a number of investigators in the United States and abroad had become interested in the possibility of transplantation of just the islet of Langerhans cells. Since it is not the entire pancreas that is at fault in diabetes but mainly the Beta cells in the islets, it seemed that transplanting these would prove more advantageous than taking the entire organ. It is true that more is known now about the role of the Alpha cells and glucagon activity, so much work remains to be done to permit manipulation of the relationship.

The procedure for isolating the Beta cells was complicated, but assiduous application by many people has overcome many of the difficulties. Generally speaking, there have been some successes in taking isolated Beta cells from one animal and putting them into a host animal at various points, but the survival of these implants has been relatively brief. While it was thought at first that the Beta cells might be resistant to the immune response that results in the rejection of implanted tissue, it was found that they were just about as prone to rejection as were any other tissues.

There is some encouraging news from various quarters concerning the rejection problem. This includes utilizing a method of implanting suspensions of these cells into the portal vein of the liver so that the islet cells implant themselves in liver tissue. Also, growing the Beta cells in tissue culture and modifying their immunological characteristics may provide a way to ensure long-term survival after implantation into the diabetic patient.

There were a couple of signs on the horizon of Beta cell transplants that have been reported and that seem to indicate that this method of providing insulin internally may yet become successful. In 1974 Dr. David W. Scharp of the Washington University School of Medicine reported that his group had implanted intact pancreatic islet cells into diabetic primates and that the animals had returned to normal or near-normal in a number of measurements. In describing this to the 1974 meeting of the American Diabetes Association, Dr. Scharp said they had transplanted donor cells via the portal vein into five diabetic rhesus monkeys. He stated that the extreme hunger, thirst, and frequency of urination in these monkeys had been reduced. He also said that their fasting blood sugars had returned to normal and that ketone bodies were significantly lowered in the blood and in the urine. The monkeys eventually rejected the islet cells, but the project did answer some questions about the ability to isolate intact islet cells and about the use of the portal vein route for transplants.

Earlier on, Drs. Walter F. Ballinger and Paul E. Lacey at Washington University reported their successful transplant of islet cells into diabetic rats. They found in the transplanted rats that urine volume, urine glucose, fasting blood sugar, and weight were normal but that there was a delayed response in an intravenous glucose tolerance test, which they were unable to explain. In reporting the work, it was said that the transplanted rats were in the normal range for all but the delayed glucose response one year after transplantation, and that, said Dr. Scharp, "is one-third of a rat's life span."

Thus it would appear that Beta cell transplant is an exciting prospect for the future, but there is still the necessity for a considerable amount of work to be done in animals before it is tried on any large group of human diabetics. However, as more and more application is made to the problems, solutions will probably be forthcoming that will make the technique successful. It almost boggles the mind, though, that a possibility exists for a method that may provide a diabetic with his own insulin, without the necessity for injection!

In the absence of complete success thus far by means of pancreas transplants or the implantation of Beta cells to provide the diabetic with his own internal supply of insulin, scientists have also been working on a mechanical means that might do the trick. Fondly called by some the "black box," this involves construction of an implantable, self-contained device that will continuously monitor glucose levels in the blood, calculate a proper insulin dose by means of a tiny computer, and then release insulin from a reservoir that is part of the equipment. And all this in a package about the size of a cardiac pacemaker or smaller, placed into a convenient point within the body!

The forerunner of this ambitious project was the artificial pancreas developed by a team of physicians and engineers in Toronto, Canada, which was tested for seven years on dogs before being turned to use on human patients. By July, 1974, it had been used to treat three diabetic patients in Toronto and five in Ulm, Germany. While the basic use of the machine is as a research tool, it was devised to make the diabetic patient more responsive to treatment when hospitalized for intensive care, coronary care, or surgery. According to statements made by A. M. Albisser, Ph.D., senior engineer of the group that designed the instrument, the patients treated in Toronto showed an unprecedented degree of control so that they were never in a situation that could be considered in any way unsatisfactory or abnormal.

At the time this artificial pancreas was described, it consisted of rather bulky machinery attached to the patient by means of tubes into his blood vessels. It contained a sensor unit through which the blood flowed and was analyzed for blood sugar level. This reading was then automatically fed into a computer, which compared it to the ''normal'' figure that had been previously entered into the computer memory bank. The computer then adjusted any deviation from the normal by controlling insulin or glucose release into the bloodstream from reservoirs of each that are part of the apparatus.

To the uninitiated it might appear simply impossible that the same thing being done by the rather massive machinery of the Toronto external artificial pancreas can be done in a device roughly the size of a package of cigarettes. However, two scientists at the opposite sides of the American continent are well on their way to accomplishing this, Dr. Samuel P. Bessman, professor and chairman of pharmacology at the University of Southern California School of Medicine in Los Angeles, and Dr. J. Stuart Soeldner, associate director of the Joslin Research Laboratory in Boston, Massachusetts.

In 1975 Dr. Bessman said that his group's research was further along than it had predicted in 1972. He reported a functioning implantable sensor that can measure glucose at body conditions, and that in 1975 the group was developing a cover for it to make it more compatible with body tissues, even though it had caused very little local reaction as it was. Dr. Bessman and a colleague, Dr. Lyell Thomas, together constructed a pump that might be called the smallest controllable pump ever made, which is capable of delivering doses of insulin from an implanted reservoir at the rate of 1/20,000 of a teaspoonful at any frequency. They designed and constructed a computer circuit that will permit the level of blood sugar to control the emission of insulin. At the functional capacity of the pump it can emit doses of insulin at the rate of 0.02 units per stroke. The entire pump, computer, power supply, and refillable insulin reservoir take up a volume of less than 60 cc. (cubic centimeters), which is about the size of a large egg. The computer is programmed to turn the pump off when the blood sugar is reduced to the low-normal range. The Bessman group has also been working on a bedside method for measuring blood sugar continuously in animals to monitor the performance of the implanted apparatus.

Dr. Soeldner has been proceeding via the development of an implantable glucose sensor/alarm that would alert the diabetic by means of a signal when his glucose level was too high or too low. This was being tested in primates in 1975. Beyond that, Dr. Soeldner has been working toward the construction of an artificial Beta cell with sensor, computer, pump, and insulin reservoir to be implanted. While the work on the sensor is essentially completed, the miniaturization of the other components was only being started late in 1975. Dr. Soeldner told the Medical News section of the *Journal of the American Medical Association* in 1973 that the artificial Beta cell would find wide use even if someone discovered an immunosuppressive drug so powerful, and so lacking in side effects, that islet cell transplants became practical on a routine basis. Finding enough donors would remain a problem, he stated, and in any case such a drug is not likely to become available soon. Furthermore, a patient with implanted Beta cells would still need to monitor his blood sugar levels to assure himself that the transplant was working properly.

There is considerable interest in studying the Beta cells themselves to determine what it is that destroys their insulin-secreting power almost completely in the juvenile-onset diabetic and permits only an ineffective response to glucose in the maturity-onset disease. There is some evidence that regeneration of the Beta cells can be stimulated by pharmacologic agents. In 1947 Beta cell neogenesis was observed to be encouraged by sulfonylureas, and there are other agents that have revived these cells to the point where they again produced normal amounts of insulin. So far, this is a promising path down which basic research might go, but there are no significant results yet.

Some authorities in the field of diabetes research feel that the work in restoring the Beta cell to normal function should be left to the geneticists. Their basic feeling is that the original fault is genetic no matter what kind of diabetes results.

One could speculate endlessly on the various areas in which research in diabetes is being conducted and on which will be the most productive. There is no doubt that the applied research that is going on—the artificial pancreas as a prime example—holds the most promise for near-term improvement in management. Yet this is closely paralleled in importance by the work with glucagon and somatostatin, which also, when moved into the clinical area, will add a new dimension to treatment and to maintenance of the diabetic in a more physiologically favorable state.

One might say that the future can only be brighter than the present and that the benefits of research, when finally applied to the patient, will change the whole face of diabetes.

What an artificial Beta cell might look like !

glucose sensor electrode   power supply   computer   pump   insulin reservoir

skin surface

8

Acute and Chronic Problems

In the light of modern medical knowledge and expertise in the treatment of diabetes, there is every reason for the diabetic to anticipate living in a fashion closely approaching the normal. While the life expectancy of a patient after onset of diabetes was 4.9 years in 1914, it rose to 18.1 years by 1970, and there is little doubt but that it is longer than that now. Concurrently, the quality of life for the diabetic has vastly improved. Whether treated by means of diet alone, through insulin therapy, or with the oral hypoglycemic agents, today's diabetic has every chance for the kind of existence that his nondiabetic friends enjoy.

The diabetic, though, however well treated, must always keep a weather eye out for his condition. He must recognize that he and his physician are attempting through external means to achieve what the nondiabetic population enjoys naturally—a satisfactory balance of metabolic activity that keeps his blood sugar within normal bounds, allowing him to live as symptom-free as possible. He is totally and irrevocably involved with his own treatment and has to be constantly alert for signs that will tell him when things might be going awry.

Since all people are differently constituted, certain standards of bodily activity are established that apply to a particular individual at any given time. There are various circumstances that can change the parameters of these in any one patient. There are acute and chronic conditions encountered in the diabetic and different situations that can alter body processes. While the basic reasons for these alterations may be somewhat similar in all people, the intensity and magnitude of the changes may vary significantly for any one of a number of causes, producing modifications in varying degree and clinical significance.

For example, there may be a gradual elevation of the blood sugar induced by overeating or underexercising, a change due to variances in the utilization patterns of the sugar. This can occur even in patients who are thought to be on an optimum dose of insulin or the oral medications, or in those being treated with diet alone. Emotional stress, infection, failure to take medication at the proper time, occurrence of disease involving body systems not even related to diabetes, are other factors that may also stimulate changes in the levels of blood sugar considered normal for that individual. The development of additional unrelated endocrine disturbances such as hypothyroidism or adrenal gland disorders or the use of such medications as cortisone, diuretics, dilantin, for example, can change the relative stability of the diabetic balance.

Some of these factors may act fairly slowly, over periods of weeks or months, producing very gradual changes in the blood sugar stability until they become obvious and are then corrected by adjustment of medication, diet, and exercise.

These situations are generally less dramatic and less threatening in their immediate effect on the patient than those causing very sudden and high rises in the blood sugar or, conversely, causing the blood sugar to dip suddenly below levels necessary for the proper functioning of body tissues, especially the brain.

Diabetic coma or ketosis is an extremely dangerous and acute state involving a great increase in the blood sugar, with a general accentuation of all of the symptoms of diabetes but compressed into an extremely short period of time, sometimes within a space of several hours. A diabetic may be getting along well and then develop a severe respiratory infection such as pneumonia. Within a short time, the patient may experience extreme thirst and increased frequency of urination and become severely dehydrated. Then, because of the nature of the basic biochemical change involved, which is related to absolute and relative deficiency of insulin, substances called ketone bodies may be produced. Ketones are fatty entities generated in great abundance in the liver and are somewhat acidic in nature, tending to bring about a generalized state of acidosis. With this comes a change in the blood chemistry, and the ketone bodies are poured out in the urine, along with certain basic substances found in the body, and the result is dehydration and a modification of the mental state of the individual. This can become so intense that it can go on to cause coma and even death if unrecognized and untreated.

The basic treatment in these cases is the use of fluid replacement to counteract the severe dehydration, and the provision of adequate amounts of insulin to help lower the abruptly elevated blood sugar. Of course, correction of the underlying cause, such as infection, is essential to proper treatment. The patient with diabetes should be able to recognize that there are certain predisposing factors that will tend to cause ketoacidosis. Infection would probably be the most common, so any type of infection from a bacterial pneumonia to a nonspecific gastroenteritis of virus nature can trigger the chain of events.

The patient may note for several days before the development of ketoacidosis that he requires a gradual increase in his insulin dose because his urine sugar is rising and he attempts to combat this through more insulin. However, there may be no warning symptoms noted at all until the situation becomes very serious medically. Extreme lethargy, fatigue, vomiting, and abdominal pain, together with the appearance of a flushed face, slow deep breathing known as air hunger, an acetone or fruity odor to the breath, plus severe and intense dehydration, are all signs that make the diagnosis apparent to an informed patient and family members.

Any diabetic can experience an episode of ketoacidosis under certain circumstances, although some people seem more resistant to its occurrence than others. The adult diabetic who is well controlled with diet or oral medication is somewhat less prone to an onset of ketosis than the insulin-dependent patient who can go into ketoacidosis much more easily. Those taking insulin should therefore certainly be alert to the possibility of this acute problem. Many juveniles will first be diagnosed as diabetics because of the intense and ferocious onset of an attack of ketoacidosis, usually following some apparently minor respiratory infection or abdominal virus attack.

Ketoacidosis was probably one of the most dangerous foes that threatened the diabetic many years ago, but it is now so well recognized and so well treated that death from it is a relative rarity. Prompt recognition and treatment is based on the awareness that it does occur as a result of fairly specific conditions, and it no longer is as life-threatening as it was.

During the past decade another state, known as hyperosmolar diabetic coma, has been defined, with signs and symptoms similar to those in ketoacidosis except that it develops more slowly, tending to be gradual and subtle in its onset. The basic physiological reason for its occurrence lies in the rate at which the ketone bodies are produced. Actually, it is felt that the patient who develops hyperosmolar coma has enough circulating insulin, either of his own making or administered by injection, to suppress the formation of the ketones. The sugar therefore rises slowly to very great levels, but the ketones do not develop, and thus the patient is less sick than in ketoacidosis. The situation can obtain over a period of from one to two weeks wherein the patient will become progressively more lethargic and dehydrated and just plain not feel well until someone notices that he is not responding and may, indeed, be in a coma. When the patient is brought to the attention of a physician, what is found is extreme dehydration, signs of great mental confusion or coma, and blood sugars that can reach 1000 mg%, which greatly exceeds those accompanying the ketoacidotic coma.

This type is often found in elderly diabetics who are confined to nursing homes or chronic disease hospitals, in whom the onset is so subtle that it may not be recognized early even by trained nursing and aide personnel. The outcome in these cases is not as good as in ketoacidosis where, because of the radical symptoms, the patient gets medical attention more quickly. In the hyperosmolar situation, the mortality may be as high as 30 percent. The treatment involves intense rehydration with adequate fluids and the use of insulin, usually in smaller quantities than is needed in ketoacidosis. Fortunately, hyperosmolar coma, which was not described much before the early 1960s, is becoming very well recognized. It is something that physicians and patients alike are now aware of, and this increased alertness should cause treatment to be started earlier, with a resultant decrease in the mortality rate.

At the other extreme from states where the blood sugar is drastically elevated is the state where its deviation from normal is in the other direction, being lowered to the point where it produces symptoms and an acute problem. This is known as hypoglycemia and occurs in patients who are taking insulin or the oral agents. It does not manifest itself in patients who are being treated by diet, and it is a state that can occur very rapidly, even within minutes, and produce a very definitive set of symptoms.

Hypoglycemia most commonly occurs when an individual takes his normal dose of insulin in the morning, then either forgets to eat lunch or has a delayed dinner and also is more active than usual. What happens is that the insulin he has injected works without being counteracted by the intake of glucose, and therefore the blood sugar is forced to extremely low levels. Because of lack of sugar the patient may develop symptoms that can involve first some lightheadedness, sweating, giddiness, inappropriate behavior, inability to think properly, confusion, trembling, and palpitations. If this continues unrecognized and is not treated immediately by an appropriate intake of sugar or administration of glucagon (which will tend to raise the sugar level), the patient can go on to convulsions and even death in some instances. One patient we know recognizes the onset of hypoglycemia by the start of a one-sided severe headache that does not respond to pain medication.

In the diabetic, when the sugar is gradually falling there may be no symptoms of hypoglycemia because the drop with concomitant reduction of insulin requirement may be reflecting improvement in management. It also may indicate abatement of unseen stress effects that may have been making the diabetes more difficult to control previously. Or it may just reflect good control of the dietary regime or better use of exercise. This sort of decrease in blood sugar, a gradual one, is not really an emergency. It is the acute drop, over a short period of time, that is the emergent state known as insulin shock, insulin reaction, or insulin hypoglycemia.

The patient should heed the importance of the regularity of his meals and his insulin doses. He should also be aware of the effects of exercise and should know the time of day when he is most vulnerable to the onset of hypoglycemia. This depends, to a large extent, on his activities and on the type of insulin he is taking. For example, NPH insulin produces most of its hypoglycemic effect about 6 to 8 hours after injection, whereas PZI insulin may act 12 to 16 hours after administration, and regular insulin may have its strongest effect 2 to 3 hours after the dose is given. The patient and the family should also be able to identify the symptoms indicating when hypoglycemia is setting in. This may vary from patient to patient and is certainly not exactly the same in every case. Once established, though, the pattern generally remains the same for an individual. Since there can be such a variation between people, the family and the patient should become acquainted with exactly what happens in a particular person.

When in doubt about any bizarre symptoms that might be indications of hypoglycemia, it is always safest for the patient to take some sugar by mouth, eat a piece of candy, or drink some fruit juice with sugar added to see if this will alleviate the complaints. It is important to realize that sugar can be present in the urine but the patient may still undergo a hypoglycemic reaction. This can happen because that urine may have been produced a few hours previously at a time when the sugar was high. The mixture of negative urine with urine containing sugar would give a positive reading even though a hypoglycemic reaction is taking place.

New York magazine in the recent past printed an article by a *New York Times* reporter who had been a diabetic for many years and, one day, when entering a subway station felt sure that he was going into insulin shock. When he reached into his pocket for the hard candy he habitually carried, he found that he had left it in another suit.

He knew the course that this reaction would take, especially the rapidity with which he would become confused and unable to communicate his predicament lucidly. He then decided that the best thing to do would be to get on the oncoming train and try to find someone in the car who would have some kind of candy or even chewing gum. Because he was quickly becoming more lethargic, less able to speak, and more disoriented, it was fortunate that the car was full of young schoolchildren going on a picnic outing. Consequently they had great numbers of such high-sugar items as candy, fruit, and sodas.

As soon as he was able to convince the people on the train that he was neither drunk nor insane, the picnic goodies came out in a hurry and he was able to take in enough high-sugar substances to overcome the reaction.

This story has a happy ending and was written primarily to show that New Yorkers, often accused of being cold and uninvolved, do care what happens to people and are willing to help someone in distress. However, it has a special message for diabetics in its description of the rapidity with which a hypoglycemic reaction can occur, and the importance of carrying some form of quick-acting sugar at all times. Implicit in the story also is that a diabetic should carry some kind of identification so that people will know what to do for him when this kind of problem occurs.

Hypoglycemia in diabetics who are taking insulin and the oral agents is fairly well understood, but there are also types of hypoglycemia that occur in people who do not have diabetes and who are not taking medications for any reason. This state is called spontaneous hypoglycemia and is of two major varieties—fasting and nonfasting. Patients whose hypoglycemia occurs spontaneously prior to eating should be investigated very carefully for various tumors that might be causing the overproduction of insulin, and also for the presence of a number of other potentially serious organic diseases. Severe liver disease, insufficient production of adrenal hormones, and pituitary disorders are serious and are the most common causes of spontaneous fasting hypoglycemia. These conditions can be diagnosed with some accuracy by the performance of glucose tolerance tests and insulin assays and can be treated by appropriate measures.

Certain patients will have all the symptoms of hypoglycemia several hours after eating; this is far more common than the fasting type and is known as reactive hypoglycemia. The exact reasons for this occurrence are not known. There is an overproduction of insulin in these patients in response to the challenge induced by a high-glucose meal so that the sugar level drops sharply, resulting in the symptoms described previously. Once this is determined, usually by a five-hour glucose tolerance test that shows the situation very clearly, it can often be treated successfully by adherence to a low-carbohydrate diet. The use of the low-carbohydrate, high-protein diet prevents the sudden release of insulin in answer to high-carbohydrate stimulus, therefore the tremendous drop in blood sugar after insulin outpouring does not occur.

Some years ago it was fashionable to ascribe all sorts of complaints of inadequacy, unhappiness, or depression to hypoglycemia and difficulty in keeping blood sugars within normal limits. It became almost a fad to make hypoglycemia the whipping boy for inadequate personalities and failure in various types of life situations. But really this was an attempt on the part of many patients to find an organic justification for what might be termed a psychological inability to cope with daily problems. There is, of course, true hypoglycemia, and this can be detected by appropriate tests. However, the majority of patients claiming to be hypoglycemic have not had this confirmed on the basis of any proper glucose tolerance test, yet they use this organic diagnosis to explain away various personality shortcomings. Unfortunately, some physicians have capitalized on these patients by treating them with a variety of medications, with differing responses. True hypoglycemia has a basis in fact and can generally be corrected by means of specific therapy. It is not found where the patient's symptoms are bizarre, without confirmatory laboratory evidence.

Hypoglycemia and ketosis are generally considered to be the two most drastic emergencies in diabetes. However, the occurrence of foot infections, though not as dramatic in the sense of quick response to treatment with resultant restoration of the patient to a normal state, is probably of equal importance in the well-being and course of the diabetic. These patients are prone to foot infections for various reasons. First of all, they may have neuropathy—nerve damage—so they do not feel trauma to the feet and lower limbs, and because of changes in the small and large blood vessels in the area, the blood supply is compromised so that healing may be retarded or prevented. In addition, the white blood cells that normally fight infection are somehow impaired in their activity, and this may not even be related to the level of blood sugar or to the degree of control of the diabetes. Finally, the culture-medium effect of sugar-rich tissue enables infections to get started and to progress sometimes at an alarming rate. The best treatment, of course, is the prevention of foot infection.

Certainly the proper type of foot care should be scrupulously followed, including correct cutting of the toenails, wearing well-fitting shoes and slippers at all times, not going barefoot, and changing socks frequently. These are fundamental methods that should be employed to prevent infections from occurring. Diabetics should see a podiatrist periodically to have their nails trimmed properly, and should use lubricants on their feet as well as skin creams to keep the skin supple and prevent it from cracking or becoming calloused, enabling infection to take hold. When infection does occur, however, the best course is to see a physician immediately because with proper treatment, including rest and the use of antibiotic medication, there is a good chance of complete healing.

Nevertheless, in patients with very poor circulation to the extremities, healing may not occur and it may be necessary to take arterial X-rays, called angiograms, to evaluate the blood supply with the thought of performing surgical reconstruction. In a fair number of patients who have progressed to this unhappy point, bypass arterial surgery can be done and may indeed be very successful in clearing up an infection.

However, in a certain percentage of patients whose severe

infection cannot be controlled by the usual conservative measures, amputation may become necessary. This is still a dread complication of diabetic infections in the lower extremities. The importance of preventive foot care in diabetics cannot be stressed too greatly. Certainly some patients, even with the best of care, will have such bad circulation that infection can occur and may eventually result in surgical amputation. But the majority of patients who must undergo an amputation are people who cut their toenails improperly and sustained an infection that was resistant to healing, or who developed a blister because of wearing new and poorly fitted shoes. In the latter case, probably the nerve damage that sometimes accompanies diabetes prevented the patient from feeling the blister, and by the time it was noticed it had spread or had started to ulcerate and could not be contained. Examining the feet often and taking good care of the lower extremities should be as seriously considered in the management of diabetes as is adhering to the prescribed diet or medication. This is definitely one situation where an ounce of prevention is worth pounds and pounds of cure.

Now, what about other acute and chronic problems facing patients who have diabetes? They can certainly be serious and may or may not be related to the disease. The other problems are certainly not as dramatic as ketoacidosis, hypoglycemia, or foot infections, but they are important to consider.

First of all, the diabetic may have to undergo surgery for any one of a number of causes. He may be injured in an automobile accident and require surgical repair, or may have appendicitis, or may have to have his gall bladder removed. Adjustments to his medication and modifications in his diet therefore have to be made prior to surgery and in the immediate postoperative period. The goal is, naturally, to keep the patient in as optimum a metabolic balance as possible. These adjustments can easily be made by most knowledgeable physicians, and there is not too much that the patient himself has to know about this. The possibility of meeting with an emergency accident is another good reason for the diabetic patient to wear some sort of identification bracelet or to carry a card describing his condition. This will enable any physician who sees the diabetic in an emergency situation to be aware of the special provisions necessary for his care. It would be wise to include the current dosage of insulin on the information card, as well as listing any other medications being taken. In addition, the name of the patient's primary physician with his address and telephone number should be set out so the emergency physician can obtain further information. It goes without saying that the patient's next of kin should be named on the card, with address and telephone number.

With most surgical procedures, the diabetic does as well as any other patient of comparable age undergoing the same sort of procedure, and well-managed diabetes presents no problems in recuperation or convalescence. The problem of wound-healing may be slightly accentuated in the diabetic, but this is not generally the case, and in most diabetics undergoing surgery the period of convalescence approximates that of most nondiabetic patients.

In another area, emotional stress has a greater effect on diabetics than on nondiabetics, with the net effect of stress being a rise in blood sugar. Its severity depends on the length and intensity of the emotional stimulus or upset. To tell the diabetic that he cannot become angry, that he shouldn't worry or permit people to get on his nerves, would be fruitless. No one who goes through life pursuing a career or relating to other people in all sorts of situations can avoid stress and strain. The diabetic must always be cognizant that things that upset him emotionally or that cause him anxiety will have an effect on the course of his control and on the level of his blood sugar. He should therefore pay particular attention to those factors which can cause severe and sometimes long-lasting fluctuations in his blood sugar.

A young woman patient of the author had been doing quite well in her diabetic control for a number of years but then, for some reason that was not apparent, she began to develop a gradual rise in the amount of sugar she was spilling into the urine as well as an increase in the levels of her fasting blood sugars. She was thoroughly studied for obscure infection, for the presence of insulin-destroying subtances in her blood, and for the appearance of other endocrine diseases that might be having an effect on the control of her disease. This continued for several months with nothing definite disclosed.

One day, when the negative results of all her tests were being evaluated and discussed, she was asked if she had any idea about what could be causing the trouble. She then released a torrent of tears and told all about the emotional stress and strain she had been undergoing in regard to problems at home with her mother, who, in effect, was refusing to allow her to grow up, to conduct her own affairs, and to live her own life. This emotional factor had not been recognized as being severely upsetting because she had always presented a very calm outward appearance and seemed to be completely free from any of the problems that beset most people.

Once this information came to light she was treated at first with tranquilizers and other psychopharmacological medication, which caused an almost immediate abrupt drop in her blood sugar so that she began having insulin reactions. Her basic diet and medication for diabetes were adjusted and she was advised to have some psychiatric counseling, which she did. Following this course, her control was reestablished and she continued to do extremely well. Thus it is not always the obvious stressful situation that may be at fault. There may be things that smolder and are kept repressed—hostilities, resentments, and worries that can exist for long periods of time, and that do not surface to become apparent—that can cause adverse effects on the control of the diabetic. These should be uncovered whenever possible and treated properly.

The diabetic who becomes pregnant evokes a number of concerns since her management and control becomes more complicated, especially in the last three months, when a great deal of attention must be paid to insulin administration and diet. It is also important to be aware that sugar in the urine of pregnant women may not be glucose, for there are other sugars that appear that are not of particular significance. Pregnancy, too, is one of the stress factors that could uncover a latent diabetic. Of all the women who produce abnormal glucose tolerance tests in pregnancy, one third may be true diabetics and continue to show diabetic glucose tolerance test results after they have delivered. In the diabetic, there may be increased rates of complications in pregnancy such as toxemia, hydramnios, and congenital defects in large babies.

In a study by J. M. Malins and M. G. Fitzgerald of the General Hospital, Birmingham, England, in 1965, it was noted that babies weighing over 10 pounds were born to 12 percent of diabetic women but to only 5 percent of nondiabetic controls observed. And, apparently, diabetes in the father has no effect on the occurrence of large babies.

Both the mother and the fetus are at considerable risk in the diabetic's pregnancy so that treatment of the diabetes and optimum timing of the delivery are crucial to a successful birth. For these reasons, most experts agree that diabetic patients should be hospitalized at about the thirty-fifth week of pregnancy and delivered no later than the thirty-seventh or thirty-eighth week. The purpose of hospitalization is to bring about maximum control of the diabetes and to obtain information essential for determining the correct time and method of delivery. Admission to hospital may be indicated at any time before the thirty-fifth week for the diabetic who has demonstrated a tendency toward preeclampsia, who has vascular problems, or who has failed in the past to deliver a live baby. The hospital might also be the best place for the diabetic pregnant woman whenever poor control occurs during her pregnancy.

Determination of the time of delivery must be made by the medical and obstetrical people working together because the hazard of delivery before the optimum time is neonatal death due to prematurity. These infants run a risk of being prone to hyaline membrane disease and must be monitored carefully. If delivery takes place after the thirty-eighth week, there is always a chance that the placenta will fail and the embryo will die *in utero*. For some reason, as yet unknown, the placenta of a diabetic can just give up its function suddenly and the baby can die literally within eight to twelve hours. Therefore considerable monitoring of the fetus and regular biochemical tests are performed to detect any signs of this happening. Of course, in the event of fetal distress as disclosed by the testing methods, or toxemia of pregnancy, there is no alternative to immediate delivery.

Regarding delivery, many elements influence the method to be employed in each case. If the patient has not previously had a cesarian section, and there are no nondiabetic obstetrical needs for such a procedure, an attempt may be made to induce labor with a pituitary extract to accomplish vaginal delivery. On the other hand, if the cervix is not soft or if labor has lasted for six to ten hours and induction fails, the cesarian section may be performed. Some authorities maintain that if induction fails twice, then the section is mandatory. During delivery, most physicians change the diabetic medication to regular insulin, which is administered as needed and as indicated by the blood and urine sugars. Great care is taken to prevent hypoglycemia in the infant or the mother immediately after delivery. In the event that the mother is taking the oral hypoglycemic agents to control her diabetes, these are usually stopped before delivery and the patient put on insulin. The oral agents' effects cross the placental boundary and may cause an upsurge in the embryo's insulin secretion, permitting it to be born hypoglycemic, with a need for close observation and perhaps administration of glucose for a time after birth. Insulin does not cross the placenta and so its use is not reflected in the fetus.

The babies of diabetic mothers are particularly prone to a vast array of complications and must be checked carefully after delivery, by a pediatrician. Respiratory distress, hyperbilirubinemia, and hypoglycemia are some of the most severe difficulties that are encountered. One authority, Dr. Henry Dolger of New York's Mt. Sinai Hospital has said that diabetics have big, flabby babies whose survival is in jeopardy.

Yet another chronic or recurring problem revolves around the entire relationship of the oral contraceptive agents, the Pill, to carbohydrate metabolism. This is not yet completely understood in the biochemical sense, but there are enough manifestations of some sort of influence to cause special attention when prescribing these drugs for diabetic women. It has been well demonstrated and well documented that it is probably the estrogen in the contraceptive pill that is responsible for the decreased glucose tolerance observed after this medication has been taken. But recent reports show that the progestin also plays an important role in this phenomenon. It would certainly seem that the oral contraceptive agents could hasten the appearance of diabetes in a potentially diabetic woman taking them, and also that there might be some deterioration in carbohydrate metabolism in nondiabetics taking the Pill. It is also interesting that some cases of persistent monilial vaginitis described by women taking the oral contraceptives may be related to impaired glucose tolerance caused by these drugs, and this possibility must also be considered when prescribing them.

The effect of menstruation on the glucose levels of diabetic women is another point of interest. As early as 1918 a report on one patient described repeated episodes of acidosis developing during menstruation, and so the adverse effects of diabetes on menstruation, and vice versa, have been known for many years. Since that time, other studies have reported poor diabetic control or insulin resistance around the time of menstruation. And many studies of carbohydrate tolerance during the menstrual cycle have confirmed the general impression that blood glucose levels of diabetics are influenced by menstruation. Diabetic control can be severely upset in some patients at that time, although it may be little changed in others. Nevertheless, the possibility of the menstrual cycle's modification of the overall diabetic control should be recognized, evaluated, and treated with the appropriate measures if necessary.

Another chronic problem, not much discussed because it is involved so inextricably with the psychological nuances of masculinity, is that of impotence in the diabetic male. It is insidious in its onset because the patient's libido remains reactive to erotic stimuli but he progressively loses his ability to have erections until the condition becomes permanent and irreversible. Impotence associated with diabetes is more common than generally realized, and studies show that it occurs in at least 50 percent of diabetic males.

Despite the frequency with which it occurs, it was only recently established that diabetic neuropathy is the basis for the impotence. In 1971, reporting in *Annals of Internal Medicine,* Dr. Max Ellenberg, clinical professor of medicine at the Mount Sinai School of Medicine and a past president of the American Diabetes Association, wrote that a neurogenic basis was suspected because potency depends on the autonomic nervous system, which is frequently affected in diabetic neuropathy.

In 1974 a group of researchers in Argentina reported in *Diabetes* (December, 1974) that the findings that Dr. Ellenberg reported were confirmed through pathological studies. The group discovered neurologic lesions of the nerve fibers that control erections in four out of five impotent diabetics on autopsy. The more pronounced abnormalities correlated with duration of illness and poor control of the disease. Since erection occurs after great engorgement with blood of the *corpora cavernosa* and *corpus spongiosa* in the penis, the penile arteries have to dilate. This is controlled by nerves, the *nervi erigentes,* which arise from the parasympathetic plexus. If these nerves suffer from diabetic neuropathy and do not stimulate the arterial dilatation, there can be no reflex of erection.

While impotence usually appears in middle-aged diabetics who have had the disease for fifteen years or more, this is not always the case. As a matter of fact, according to Dr. Ellenberg, impotence can be the initial presenting manifestation of diabetes. If a man of forty or forty-five who has previously been potent is losing his erections and the cause is not clearly psychogenic, the physician must suspect the possibility of diabetes.

A determination has to be made as to whether the impotence is the result of diabetic neuropathy and therefore is permanent, or is due to some psychogenic cause. In the case of the diabetic, impotence has a gradual onset and libido is retained. In impotence from psychological cause, the state usually occurs suddenly, and libido is lost as well, but there are periods of remission. One factor in the onset of diabetic impotence is that the patient is usually aware of the possibility of its occurrence, so he becomes anxious and adds a psychological component to the organic base. Counseling the diabetic whose impotence has been ruled absolutely to be the result of his disease can be tricky. However, since sexual virility is so intricately tied in with masculinity and a man's view of himself, the impotent diabetic is usually relieved to find that his condition is due to a factor over which he has no control. This seems to be more acceptable than thinking it results from some inadequacy as a male.

Conventional sexual intercourse, the patient should understand, is not the only expression of sexuality; there is more than one way in which a couple can satisfy each other. This, also, is a delicate subject, and the physician has to know his patient extremely well before he suggests the alternatives of manual or oral sex as a substitute for genital-to-genital intercourse.

While Dr. Robert C. Kolodny, director of the endocrine program at the Reproductive Biology Research Foundation in

St. Louis, published a study in *Diabetes* in August, 1971, that indicated that diabetic women reported more nonorgasmic experience than did nondiabetic women, other researchers do not agree. Dr. Ellenberg, for one, found no changes in the sexual response in the female diabetic up to this point in his research.

There are both acute and chronic problems in diabetes, and they should be respected for the influence they may have on the course of the patient's life. There are few, however, where good control and good management cannot help but reduce their effects so that the diabetic can adjust to them. The diabetic's motto should be: respect, yes; fear and trembling, no!

9

Complications of Diabetes

The diabetic in today's world can enjoy enough freedom of activity to relish both the quantity and quality of life. With modern treatment methods and some freedom of diet now that a relaxation of rigid control has been accepted as sound practice, it is often difficult to distinguish the diabetic from the nondiabetic in normal social intercourse. True, the diabetic is not absolutely free from concern over his metabolic regulation. He must still be aware of the balance in his medication, diet, and activity, but in the short run, on a day-to-day basis, one can accommodate to the disease without too much difficulty.

And as medical science progresses, when the ideas and methods now in the laboratory are phased into clinical realities, there surely will come a greater emancipation of the diabetic from the stresses and strains of coping with the disease.

It is in the long run that the diabetic is not yet out of the woods. That the disease itself has a cumulative degenerative effect on various body organs, systems, and processes is still true. That medical science has not yet been able to determine the cause of the eventual damage wrought by diabetes or the mechanism through which it transpires is also a fact. Probably the fundamental reason for this lack of knowledge is that no one has yet identified the basic defect that results in diabetes. Disclosure of what can go wrong, yes; bits and pieces of the biochemical puzzle with signs pointing in various directions, yes; but none adding up to a clear-cut answer to the question: why does the diabetic have an inability to metabolize carbohydrates normally?

Also, medical science has not as yet been able to define the exact reason or reasons for the devastating effect diabetes has in the tissues where it can do the most damage.

In testimony given before the United States Senate Subcommittee on Health of the Committee on Labor and Public Welfare in 1973, Dr. James B. Field, professor of medicine at the University of Pittsburgh School of Medicine, stated:

> Before insulin, diabetic coma caused about 50 percent of the deaths in diabetic patients, but it now accounts for less than five percent of diabetic deaths.
>
> In contrast to this impressive reduction in mortality due to diabetic coma, there has been a progressive increase in disability and deaths due to the vascular complications of diabetes. Today, about 70 percent of diabetic patients die from the degenerative vascular complications which affect the blood vessels of the heart, brain, extremities, eyes, kidneys and nerves. It is these changes which are responsible for the strikingly increased incidence of heart attacks, strokes, blindness, kidney failure, amputation and obstetrical mishaps in the diabetic. Before insulin, diabetic patients usually did not survive long enough to develop these vascular complications.

The most characteristic finding in diabetes when tissue is examined under the microscope is a thickening of the so-called basement membrane portions of the small blood vessels throughout the body. This is called microangiopathy, and it may result in modifying the normal function of these blood vessels so that the organs they serve do not perform in a proper manner. This occurs primarily in the eyes, in the kidneys, and in the nerves.

In the eye there is a change called a microaneurysm, which the physician sees as a small red dot during an eye examination. These small red dots in the blood vessels of the retina, the back of the eyeball, occasionally progress to form small, fragile new vessels growing out from the back of the eye. These intrude into the liquid substance of the eye and occasionally form hemorrhages, which can further create fibrous connections between the liquid of the eye and the retina, resulting in retinal detachment and blindness. Cataracts are also found with great frequency in diabetics. But within the eye itself, it is the aneurysms and their outgrowth that cause the greatest difficulty.

Frequent and regular eye examinations are essential in the care of the diabetic, for these changes can be spotted quite early with the ophthalmoscope. In fact, there is now a new technique based on the injection of a fluorescent dye, called fluorescein, which can pick up diabetic eye changes even before they become apparent by means of conventional eye examination. The cause of these particular changes in the eye, as indeed with all changes of diabetic small-blood-vessel disease, is difficult to define, but it is known that the longer the patient has diabetes, the more likely it is that these changes will occur.

As far as the eye changes are concerned, it is difficult to evaluate methods of treatment with any degree of certainty. Some of these eye changes tend to come and go spontaneously over a period of years and do not always have an inexorable, progressive course leading to the loss of vision.

Sometimes even the most severe disease that affects vision in a cumulative deteriorating way can remit and tend to reverse itself. For certain patients in whom there is a progressive decrease in visual acuity that is relentless and without remission, there are a number of maneuvers that can be tried in attempts to prevent further loss of sight.

One of the earliest of these was to try to destroy the pituitary gland. It was noticed in the early 1950s that a pregnant woman, a diabetic with severe, proliferative, and progressive retinal changes, following the delivery of her child had what is called a postpartum necrosis of the pituitary gland. In effect, her pituitary was destroyed by a blood clot, and subsequent to this, her vision began to improve a great deal. Based on this rather fortuitous observation, investigators felt that if the pituitary gland could be interfered with so it would become inoperative in patients with degenerative retinal disease, a beneficial effect would follow. A large number of studies of this nature were attempted, and there was improvement in many patients.

However, the various surgical techniques of pituitary removal had a great number of complications associated with them, and also the process of pituitary destruction caused many other changes throughout the body, so that the general medical management of these patients was very difficult. The pituitary is known as the "master gland," and so cessation of its functioning influenced the actions of other glands. For example, after its removal there were problems with the thyroid gland, with the adrenal glands, and with sexual activity, with the result that a great many medications and different types of treatment had to be applied to try to restore functions of the pituitary that would not adversely affect the vision of the patient. This mode of therapy for diabetic eye problems is rarely used at present, but there are some patients who might benefit from it.

Progressive retinal change is now treated with photocoagulation attempts with laser beams and the white-light photocoagulator. In these techniques laser lights of various kinds, such as a ruby or green laser, or argon laser, is used to burn out and destroy the little, fragile new blood vessels that grow into the vitreous fluid of the eye and can hemorrhage. The technique also tends to seal down the retina on the tissue behind it so that, in case of bleeding, the likelihood of retinal detachment will be greatly reduced. Photocoagulation has been used in a great many patients, and the results are still being fully evaluated. In certain cases it certainly has seemed to preserve failing vision, although restoration of sight has been very rare. However, there is a large continuing study going on throughout the United States at this time, attempting to evaluate the true place of this procedure in the alleviation of diabetic retinopathy. One of the great problems in the assessment is that, even in the very severe cases, there is some tendency in these patients for the condition to wax and wane, independently of anything that is done in these patients. Thus further statements regarding the real value of this treatment will have to wait for the completion of the study and the compilation of the data therefrom.

One of the newest developments in the treatment of retinopathy involves the use of somatostatin. Its action interferes with human growth hormone secreted by the pituitary gland, which is thought in large measure to contribute to the development of retinal changes. Since somatostatin blocks the effects of growth hormone, its application may prove to be, in the future, a nonoperative type of therapy that offers promise since it will ward off the changes in the small blood vessels by acting on the hormone that helps to produce them.

A relatively new surgical procedure, called total vitrectomy, has been found effective in some cases where the hemorrhaging has caused dense membranes and opacities to form in the liquid substance of the eye. With a tiny penlike instrument called the Roto-Extractor, in conjunction with a microscope, the surgeon enters the eye through a small incision. With a rotating, cutting action he removes the opacities by suction, simultaneously replacing the vitreous fluid with a saline solution. In this way, transparency is returned to the fluid in the eyeball so that the light rays going into the eye reach the retina. The procedure is suitable only in patients whose eyes have retained some function.

In the kidney, changes of the basement membrane of the glomerulus, or filtering element, tends to produce a poorly functioning filter, with resultant leakage of protein and ultimate deterioration and destruction of the kidney activity, and with the outcome seen as renal insufficiency and uremia.

Diabetics are also more prone for a variety of reasons to suffer urinary tract infections such as cystitis and pyelonephritis. But the eventual destructive portion of the diabetes syndrome in the kidney is the onset of diabetic renal disease with uremia. The treatment of this, as in the conventional treatment of most cases of renal insufficiency, is with diet, prevention of infection, and, more recently, dialysis aiming toward kidney transplant. The use of dialysis has become more and more popular in the past few years as the methods have improved and as diabetics have been recognized as suitable candidates for donor kidneys. There have been between twenty and thirty transplants done since 1973 in various centers throughout the United States, with quite good results in restoration of kidney function. In several cases, some of the eye changes that occurred along with the kidney failures seemed to regress after the transplantation. Occasionally kidney and pancreas transplants have been done at the same time, although the success rate with pancreas transplantation has been very poor.

In the nervous system there are a great many things that can occur as a result of the late complications of diabetes. These all seem to be based on a demyelinization, or loss of the insulating material of the nerves, following interference with the small blood vessels that nourish the nerves. The most common problem is the sensation of pins and needles in the hands and feet known as peripheral neuropathy. This may vary and produce a very severe sensation called diabetic amyotrophy, which usually occurs in the thigh on one side or the other, is very often much more painful than the usual diabetic neuropathy, and is sometimes accompanied by actual loss of muscle substance or atrophy of the muscle. In addition, there may be visceral neuropathy, which can produce impotence, diarrhea, and various changes in bladder function.

In the eye a variety of nerve changes can be found, which may produce different kinds of drooping of the eyelids and double vision.

There is no specific treatment for any of the changes due to neuropathy. The common type of peripheral neuropathy in the lower extremities will very often gradually improve even after one or two years of manifestation, tending to lessen or sometimes completely disappear. The pain of diabetic amyotrophy also seems to clear spontaneously in some people. It is known that the neuropathic eye changes in diabetes will very often repair themselves after six to eight weeks. In certain patients, medications such as Dilantin and Tegretol have been used, but the results are very inconsistent and really not to be recommended in all cases.

In addition to these specific small-blood-vessel changes, there is an increased incidence of larger-vessel disease in diabetes. The diabetic has approximately five times the amount of coronary artery disease as the nondiabetic, and certainly an increased number of strokes and peripheral arteriosclerosis when compared to the nondiabetic counterpart of the same age and sex. The reasons for this are not clear, unfortunately. There seems to be some relationship of the dietary fats to arteriosclerosis, and since diabetics very often tend to have elevated cholesterol and triglyceride levels, this may be at the root of their increased arteriosclerosis. It is a fact that the diet of diabetics for years has been somewhat restricted in carbohydrate, with fat being added to make up the caloric difference. Now that the American Diabetes Association has suggested a relaxation of the restriction on carbohydrate with a concurrent decrease in the amount of fat, perhaps this will combat the development of severe, early, and premature arteriosclerotic degeneration in the diabetic. In this, time alone will tell.

Another complication in patients who are taking insulin is the development of subcutaneous atrophy. This is the occurrence of changes in the tissue under the skin at the sites of repeated insulin injection. The reasons for these depressions and the thinning of tissue is not known, but it presents no great problem, other than a cosmetic one, especially in these days of bikinis, that might show up what are considered blemishes. Theoretically there can also be some erratic absorption of insulin, making for poor control, if these areas are used repeatedly for injection sites. Fortunately the development and use of U-100 insulin has tended to mitigate the problem in good measure. Injection of this particular insulin under the skin usually does not cause atrophy; in fact, it has been shown that when U-100 insulin is injected into atrophic areas, they are very often restored to normal appearance within several months.

Another problem sometimes seen is allergy to insulin. This is quite a rare condition and is often due to a beef or pork product that is found as a contaminant in commercial insulin. The manifestations of this vary from hives or itching to an occasional very severe reaction called anaphylaxis, which requires the attention of a physician. This can be a generalized allergic reaction with hives and sometimes swelling of the larynx, accompanied by difficulty in breathing. Considering the number of patients who are taking doses and doses of insulin every day, the incidence of this kind of allergic reaction is extremely rare. Sometimes the treatment of insulin allergy is merely switching to another brand or to a product derived from pure beef, pure pork, or pure fish source, rather than the mixture of beef and pork insulin from which most of the commercial product is made. There are also a number of special insulins obtainable from pharmaceutical companies that tend to mitigate against insulin allergy.

Accompanying insulin allergy can be the development of antibodies to insulin and what is known as insulin resistance. This is said to occur when a patient requires over 200 units a day to keep himself controlled, over a period of at least two weeks, and in the absence of any infection or other situation that might be an obvious cause of increased insulin demand. This is felt to occur because antibodies are made by the individuals who are taking insulin, as a response to its administration, and usually they are not significant. But in some people very high amounts of antibodies are produced that tend to bind the insulin and make it ineffective. Insulin resistance, fortunately, is a self-limiting state that can clear up within several months, but it is often necessary to treat it in order to keep the sugar levels under control during the period it is present. There are a variety of ways in which this can be done, and there are certain special insulins obtainable from pharmaceutical companies that are effective in treating this condition. Occasionally, small doses of cortisone are used, paradoxical as it may seem, to try to block the formation of antibodies and to restore the insulin function to normal.

There has long been tremendous speculation among medical scientists concerning the development of microangiopathy and its effects in the eyes, kidneys, and extremities, as well as the influence on the larger arteries. Probably the only thing on which there is general agreement is that the process is poorly understood. It has been established that the most important factor in the genesis of vascular disease in diabetics is time. The longer the disease is present, the greater the chance of vascular complications appearing, although there is increasing evidence to suggest that the development of microangiopathy may be prevented or retarded by the institution of good control.

10

The Diabetic in a Nondiabetic World

The diabetic does not live in a vacuum, nor does he live in a world where a majority of people have his problem. He does live among individuals who may be sympathetic about his disease but may not necessarily understand all of its implications. They may, therefore, make some allowances that are primary to the diabetic's comfort and well-being, but they may also be either ignorant of or indifferent to other things pertinent to the diabetic state that can affect the patient. It therefore falls to the diabetic to make those adjustments which will permit him to function well in a nondiabetic world. In having the disease one does not close out aspirations for a successful career, for normal social intercourse, and for a fulfilling family life. Quite to the contrary, the diabetic wants and needs to enjoy the same freedom in life as does his nondiabetic counterparts.

While people react in different ways to the news that they have the disease, there appear to be some common psychological responses that occur. First, of course, is the sense of shock and of disbelief that this could happen, as well as a denial of the diagnosis, usually accompanied by a basic feeling of "Why me?" Also occurring is a nagging feeling of chagrin and even some shame at this untoward turn of events.

When the understanding finally sinks in, the average maturity-onset diabetic is almost overcome by despair at the knowledge that he is now host to a condition that will stay with him the rest of his life. He also realizes, if he has heard anything at all about the disease, that there are complications that may follow that could make his life very difficult and unpleasant sometime in the future. He has an overwhelming desire to hide the fact of his disease from friends, neighbors, and employer because of the sense of shame and the subtle conviction that it is somehow "unclean."

The reaction of one fifty-two-year-old man diagnosed as a maturity-onset diabetic could be construed as typical of some of the psychological factors and reactions that make their appearances. This is a man who holds a very demanding, complicated, and stressful job, has a tremendously varied number of outside interests, owned a sport-fishing boat as a hobby, was extremely active in a high-ranking position in the active armed forces reserve, and literally "had not been sick a day in his life" with any organic disease.

Soon after a particularly severe bout of the grippe or flu he began to notice that he was always extremely thirsty and had an almost constant desire to urinate, doing so copiously about every hour or so. He also noted that he was very tired, unenthusiastic, and irritable, the last coming as a surprise because he had always been of an even, reasonably tranquil disposition. Accompanying these symptoms was a steady loss in weight despite eating a great amount in an effort to stem the tide. After a loss of thirty-five pounds over a three-month period and the comment by a neighbor in the boat slip next to his at the marina of "Are you trying to be the thinnest man in the cemetery?" he saw his physician. A two-hour postprandial blood sugar test revealed a finding well in the diabetic range, confirming the other symptoms of polyuria, polydipsia, and chronic fatigue.

Well, this elicited the familiar reactions of disbelief, shock, amazement, and despair coupled with the feeling of shame, all known to physicians whose practices are heavily concerned with diabetics. The patient could not believe that the diagnosis was firm and unquestionable, demanding that tests be repeated for absolute verification. He was unconsolable and depressed to a marked degree. He complained bitterly to his wife about this "horrible" development at a point in his life when a modicum of success in his profession was at hand, fearing that he would progress to such a debilitated state that he would not be able to cope with his responsibilities. In possession of an educated layman's knowledge of medicine, he was firmly convinced that he would fall ill to all of the complications of diabetes and that the process of "rotting away" inside had already started. He was sure that this would shorten his life, while limiting his activities because of inability to muster the energy or desire to continue them. The very thought of taking insulin and "being tied to a needle" absolutely appalled him, and he refused even to consider that mode of therapy.

His physician prescribed a combination of the oral agents, and these worked fairly well for a time, but subsequent examinations and blood sugar tests indicated that his control was not optimum. The patient, who stands 6 feet 1 inch tall, sustained a final weight loss of 40 pounds from a pre-disease weight of 185, not really in the obese category. His weight had stabilized at 145 pounds, he was still very thirsty, urinating frequently, and still rather listless and chronically fatigued.

Finally, after considerable urging from his wife and strong assurances from his physician, he agreed to try insulin and almost immediately improved in all aspects of his disease. Today he functions very well in all of his responsibilities, maintains an acceptable blood sugar level, and keeps his weight at about 160 pounds.

Psychologically, though, at first he was what might literally be called a disaster. He partially withdrew from friends and business colleagues alike. He refused to allow his wife to tell anyone in her family, nor did he tell anyone in his immediate family about his disease. So fearful was he that friends would find out about it, he would often eat carbohydrate-rich food at dinner parties rather than refuse them and thus appear strange or unusual. When people asked about his weight loss he would hint that it was the result of a strict diet, or he would almost brag that he had the kind of metabolism that would allow him food excesses not permitted other people who wanted to keep their weight down. And he kept the fact of his diabetes from his employer because of the shame he felt about it and the fear that he might be considered less capable because of the disease.

Over the years his acceptance of diabetes and his accommodation to it has improved, helped by the counseling, advice, and support given him by his wife and his physician. He readily admits, when asked, or even on occasion offers the information that he is a diabetic. In company, he refuses foods that would be off his diet without feeling that he is grotesque in any way.

Now, this total syndrome of reaction took place in a mature, well-adjusted adult who is educated, intelligent, sophisticated, and knowledgeable in matters of health. Fortunately he was able to come to peace with the fact of his disease, finally, without too much psychological damage. Since this kind of response is not unusual in chronic diseases, there are other people who do not do as well and who must seek professional counseling. They need help in finding a way of living with the disease; they need assistance in viewing the disease and themselves in the kind of perspective that will allow them to live productively without considering themselves health cripples. It is rare that an individual who is diagnosed as diabetic does not evidence some form of this kind of reaction.

In the juvenile-onset form of diabetes, the psychological factors play a most important role. In this type the need for insulin is immediate. There is also vital necessity for good management at the very outset because of the constant threat of ketoacidosis and possible coma. In addition, the child can go from bounding good health to severe and fulminating diabetes in a matter of days, perhaps even hours, providing no time for preparation to accept the condition.

To the youngster a rigid, measured, controlled way of life is anathema because of the youthful desire to attain a reasonable amount of independence and freedom from restrictive measures. Diabetes, of course, imposes limitations on one's way of life with which the child, who is normally inclined to be rebellious, finds it difficult to cope. It has the effect of setting him aside from his peer group so that the natural development process that makes him a member of the "gang" is inhibited, causing great resentment. It also has the effect of having his parents carefully and intensively oversee all of his activities to ensure compliance with the prescribed regime, another source of resentment and rebellion.

This dissatisfaction with being different and with needing to keep to a well-ordered regimen may, in the juvenile, manifest itself in various ways. The child may fake the results of urine tests, may skip insulin injections, or may abdicate the control so completely that the parent must take over. The child may act out his resentments in other ways, too, because he has the same feelings of guilt and shame about the disease condition that are felt by the adult diabetic. The same "Why me?" question is asked by the child over and over, and the same desire to hide the condition is experienced by the juvenile as it is by the adult.

The teen-ager may become extremely depressed and may

feel that the disease came to him as a punishment for some imagined sin. Unfortunately, the guilt engendered by this attitude is often shared by the parents, a common phenomenon in many childhood health problems—that the disease occurred because of some deficiency on the part of the parents. This can lead to overprotectiveness by the parents, which also causes resentment on the part of the child. There is little doubt that all illness affects personality, and a chronic illness in a teen-ager often intensifies any aberration in personality that may have preceded the disease condition. In addition, the teen-ager has a remarkable preoccupation with food, often affecting some very exotic eating habits, involved usually with just the kind of food forbidden to diabetics. The recent trend toward relaxation of some dietary restrictions on carbohydrates has helped the juvenile diabetic since it does permit some of the same kind of snacks his friends indulge in, but he is still not completely free in his diet.

The teen-ager is also known for his concern over self-image, and any stigmata that set him aside from his fellows cannot be abided with good grace and complete acceptance.

To add to the problems, diabetes in youngsters is very often influenced by the fact that they are growing rapidly, with a number of other hormones involved in the process, and that they are maturing sexually. All these factors tend to make their diabetes somewhat unstable and to bounce them from periods of high blood sugars into low blood sugars. Piled atop of this is the burden imposed by the necessity to keep to a fairly regular regime, and thus it can easily be seen that many youngsters are called labile or unstable juvenile diabetics. This situation is sometimes called "brittle diabetes."

The dictatorial or threatening approach to the management of the teen-aged diabetic is one that is probably the least effective. It is difficult in some young diabetics for the parents, or the physician, to take an extremely hard line because of the danger of stigmatizing them further and alienating them from their peers, but certainly they cannot be abandoned to an absolutely permissive diet with the resulting wide swings and fluctuations in the blood sugar, which are felt to be harmful over the long run. However, to this age group, the more orders given and the more threats made, the greater the tendency to assert oneself in defiance.

Instead, the youngster and the parents should be educated about the disease and the ways in which treatment can help without disrupting the normal life of the child or the family. The patient and the family should also be made aware that the disease's cause is basically genetic in origin and its mode of transmission is not truly known. Probably the only way to ensure remaining free from diabetes would be to choose one's ancestors carefully. If the young patient strays from the prescribed regime from time to time, this should be expected and the child should not be criticized too severely. If possible, convince him that part of the process of growing up is acceptance of responsibility for his behavior. Try to make him understand that one of the signs of maturity, with resultant consideration as an adult, is the ability to accept an unchangeable situation and to live with it in the best manner possible.

Of course, among the best means of convincing a child to follow the proper diet and medication routine is to have him see that there are other youngsters in the same situation. One way of doing this is to send him to a camp for diabetic children where he will be thrown in with peers who have the same medical problem, and where the atmosphere is cheerful, active, and fun-filled. If the child has been overly dependent on his parents to manage his disease, he will find at camp that his friends are doing their own thing and he will probably want to emulate them so that he will truly be one of the crowd. One such camp is Camp NYDA, operated by the New York Diabetes Association. Located in Burlingham, New York, on a campus of several hundred acres of woods and lake, Camp NYDA takes children from the ages of six through fourteen. Each child attends for a four-week period, and no child is refused admission because of inability to pay the full fee. Every camper, regardless of age, learns to give his or her own insulin, to make the daily urine tests, to understand diet, and to have the consistent daily exercise essential to health. And the activities are as well rounded as those found in any other children's camp. Many diabetes associations also operate similar camps, and they are really a marvelous and constructive experience for the diabetic child.

If these means fail to instill in the child a willingness to cope with his disease, then there is nothing left for both the patient and the parent but to seek professional counseling. The first resource here should be the primary physician and his advice. If this turns out to be ineffective, then the recourse is to the social worker, guidance counselor, psychologist, or psychiatrist to uncover the hidden factors that may be mitigating against successful management of the teen-aged patient. Very often, if the parent can be convinced to make his peace with the fact of a diabetic child, the young patient himself will need but brief psychotherapy. Hopefully, the end result of such counseling or guidance is the acceptance by the young patient of self-responsibility, increased freedom from dependence on the family, and a greater role in making the decisions that affect him.

Equally, in the maturing process, the school environment is one that should be supportive of the diabetic without stifling him. Guidance should be available so that the choice of vocation is one that would not be self-limiting because of the diabetes.

It would be ideal in this somewhat less than ideal world were people to understand fully the meaning of chronic disease so that they would be sympathetic and empathetic to the patient without being overweeningly solicitous. What the diabetic needs from friends and associates is the realization that he is not unduly handicapped by his disease. He can live even as they do, and he knows how he ought to work, eat, sleep, exercise, and participate in social activities. What he does not need is having someone preempt his knowledge or denigrate the importance of what he knows is vital to his welfare. Of course, the diabetic's family and friends need to know the signs and symptoms of insulin reaction as well as ketoacidosis, and should know what to do should the diabetic fall into either state.

As family, friends, and associates should understand the needs of the diabetic, so the patient has to recognize his responsibility to others. He should carry identification stating that he is a diabetic, giving his name, address, medication dosage, physician's name, address, and telephone number, and the name, address and telephone number of the person to be notified in case of emergency. The card should also contain a description of emergency measures under different circumstances: for example, that if the person is behaving in an irrational manner he is probably undergoing an insulin reaction and should be given something with a high sugar content.

There are organizations that have these cards already printed, and some that provide identification bracelets or necklaces that indicate a person's illness. One of these is Medic-Alert Foundation International, Turlock, California, 95380; another is the American Medical Association at 535 North Dearborn Street, Chicago, Illinois, 60610.

In the normal course of life, the diabetic will want to travel either on vacation or on business, and there is no reason why he should not do so. If going to a foreign country, it would be wise to be able to say in the particular language, "I am a diabetic," and "I need some sugar or something sweet," and "Get me a doctor." In addition to the identification card described earlier, patients who are taking insulin should carry a note from their doctor saying that they are diabetic and they require insulin by injection. This will provide the reason for carrying syringes and needles through customs and will prevent a great deal of trouble in getting in and out of foreign countries. In addition to whatever habitual type of insulin the patient uses, it would be a good idea to take along some regular, quick-acting insulin in case of any emergency. Insulin does not have to be refrigerated but should be kept in a cool place and should be carried in an onboard bag on the aircraft so that it can be close by. It is not wise to keep the insulin in the luggage going into the baggage compartment, since it may freeze and thaw, changing its potency in the process.

In traveling, the diabetic should continue his practice of carrying candy or lump sugar with him in case there is a delay in meal service or a late landing that interferes with regular meal time. Certain problems may be associated with traveling east or west across a number of time zones, and the doctor can advise about adjustment of insulin dose. Care should be taken not to overdo activity without adjusting the insulin dose or taking in some extra carbohydrate to avoid hypoglycemia. Other precautions involve wearing the proper shoes while sightseeing and following instructions regarding food and water in the foreign lands. Otherwise, the diabetic can enjoy the same travel as does his nondiabetic counterpart.

As more and more is known about the disease, and as more and more people fall ill with it, diabetics will be treated like normal humans in regard to insurance and employment. Better control and management have lengthened the lives of diabetics so that some insurance companies will now issue policies on them whereas in the past this was well-nigh impossible. True, because it does have an effect on life-span, there may be an increased premium required, but the diabetic is not necessarily foreclosed completely from obtaining insurance. The American Diabetes Association at 1 West Forty-eighth Street, New York, N.Y. 10020, can advise on this matter.

The diabetic who is controlled by diet alone should have no difficulty in obtaining any kind of employment. Those on oral medications as well will usually find few limitations in jobs. It is the insulin-dependent diabetic who might be precluded from certain kinds of work. Since the possibility of a hypoglycemic reaction is always present in these patients, it is better that they not aim at being airline pilots, bus or taxi drivers, or controllers of heavy equipment. The insulin-requiring diabetic in good control should otherwise find little in the way of employment closed to him. Formerly, in the hiring of diabetics, employers were concerned over insulin shock, absenteeism, and higher premiums on compensation and group insurance. These objections have, however, mostly been overcome, basically because of the performance of diabetics in various job situations. Where there is a good industrial medical program, where the diabetic is under good control and well cared for, and where the company exercises optimum job placement, the diabetic is as productive a worker as the nondiabetic, even taking into account the attendance records of each.

Because the diabetic, to maintain a well-ordered, smooth existence, has to be intimately involved in his treatment, he is inclined to become rather intensely occupied with self. This is natural, and the people with whom the diabetic comes into contact on a regular basis should respect his concern. He should not, though, be permitted to carry this to the point where he thinks he is almost crippled by his disease, nor should his friends have to treat him as though he were made of glass.

By all counts, the diabetic in a normal world should be able to live the productive and satisfying existence he enjoyed before the diagnosis was made. Through good control of his blood sugar he can possibly remain free of the worst results of the well-known diabetic complications. Also through good control, his day-to-day energies can remain at a high level and he does not have to be plagued by chronic fatigue, listlessness, and lack of enthusiasm, which are characteristic of the diabetic under poor management.

The diabetic must never forget that the best judge of his

condition is himself and that he is in control of his own destiny where the diabetes is involved. No one else can help him, no one else can control him, no one else can ensure that his condition will be stable. He must do it himself.

11

What the Future Holds

As diabetes mellitus is viewed in all its manifestations, possible causes, worldwide occurrence, and short- and long-term effects, the unmistakable conclusion is that the longer and more intensely it is studied, the more complex and mysterious it appears. What was long considered to be a simple disease caused by a lack of insulin is now known to be an illness whose activity has an effect on almost every area of the body. Not only that, but solid scientific evidence is at hand to support the concept that diabetes mellitus is considerably more than merely a lack of insulin but is a multihormonal disturbance.

In addition, the old beliefs concerning susceptibility to the disease on the part of individuals and racial groups have had to be discarded because diabetes mellitus appears now in all parts of the world, and in cultures ranging from the most primitive to the most highly developed. Truly, it is a baffling public health problem. Truly, medical scientists are literally finding it difficult to determine even a starting point for the studies that may ultimately pinpoint the causative factor or factors that result in the classic diabetes manifestation—the inability to metabolize carbohydrates normally.

One fact has emerged crystal clear out of the fog of basic ignorance about diabetes mellitus. No one in any civilization in any corner of the world is safe from the disease. As an accompaniment to this reality is another that states that the reasons for diabetes occurring in places where historically it had never been a problem are not yet understood. Studies have been made of people who have changed their life-styles as well as their diets and have become diabetic, and some investigations have been made into the socioeconomic and psychological factors obtaining when a previously rural population becomes urban, with an accompanying rise in the incidence of diabetes among it. Some of the findings about these kinds of changes and their effects on susceptibility appear valid, and others seem inconclusive. One might say that this is the story of diabetes from the earliest days of recorded medical history!

At this moment there do not even exist solid data concerning the true incidence of the disease, because a sweeping health survey has not been made in recent years. The last comprehensive effort to determine the number of diabetics in the United States was made in 1965–66, and any data that would be relevant now have to be extrapolated from the information compiled then. And this can only be done on a statistical basis, not on actual up-to-date evidence.

Also, it is just recently that enough interest in this mounting menace to health was expressed in the Congress of the United States to stimulate that body to pass the National Diabetes Research and Education Act, Public Law 93–354, which provides specific financial support for research, as well as establishing a National Commission on Diabetes. This group, comprised of four lay persons (two of them either diabetics or who had diabetic children), six physicians and/or scientists, and the seven directors of the involved National Institutes of Health, was appointed in March, 1975. The commission was charged with the following tasks:

1. Survey every aspect of the diabetes problem, including the research areas that need more attention;
2. formulate a long-range plan toward the solution; and
3. make budgetary recommendations and report back to Congress with these and any other recommendations.

The commission was also charged with accomplishing this project within one year of appointment. In carrying out the bill's provisions concerning the establishment and expansion of diabetes research and training centers, the National Institute of Arthritis, Metabolism, and Digestive Diseases has created four of these. The first was set up in Nashville, Tennessee; and others followed in Seattle, Washington; Chicago, Illinois; and Charlotte, North Carolina. More centers will be established as funds become available.

The Commission made its report in December, 1975, well ahead of its March, 1976 deadline. It said, in part, ". . . Diabetes and its complications are responsible for more than 300,000 deaths annually, raising diabetes to the third ranking cause of death—behind cardiovascular (heart) disease and cancer. . ."

It also stated that at the current rate of increase, the number of Americans with diabetes will double every 15 years.

The Commission's proposal for coping with the disease involves a long-range plan of broadened research, education and control programs. It requests a tripling of Federal research spending on diabetes in the next four years. The total Federal research spending on diabetes from 1976 through

1980 would be about $548 million under the Commission plan.

The Commission proposed four major items: increased research, increased manpower training, increased diabetes health care, education and control programs, and the establishment of a diabetes advisory board to evaluate progress and give advice to the Government and a yearly report to Congress and the Administration.

Senators Richard S. Schweiker of Pennsylvania and Gail W. McGee of Wyoming are two legislators strongly advocating a greater concern for a major assault on diabetes. Diabetes is thus added to those major disease categories that have been singled out for special attention/ in recent years. Cancer and heart disease already have gained increased research funding, as have kidney dialysis and transplantation, the latter two now classified as treatment for which the Federal Government will reimburse costs to patients.

Before the passage of the diabetes legislation, research into the disease was supported meagerly and sporadically, and this in the face of an illness that costs the country more than $5 billion annually. This neglect might stem from the lack of complete understanding of diabetes, ignorance of its menacing capabilities, unawareness of its magnitude in the population and of its ultimate effects in those suffering from the disease. The diabetic does not evidence any stigmata to indicate the disease, and his condition is visible to his associates only if he discloses it or is one of those whose disease progresses to the point where the complications become apparent.

It is an encouraging sign to those most concerned about diabetes and its consequences that at least it is now seen as a formidable threat by the lay community as well as by the medical profession. This recognition had to be the first step in addressing the problem. Until realization of the danger of diabetes, and its increased incidence, was clear to people in general, no substantial effort could be mounted against it.

There is every reason to believe that as more and more people become diabetic and their friends, relatives, and business associates are aware of this, there will be a heightened concern about the disease as an enemy that must be conquered. And when public opinion, stimulated by knowledge, is accompanied by public pressure, the war on diabetes will certainly increase in intensity.

There is probably little doubt that the interest in diabetes on the part of medical researchers arises as much from the desire to solve a knotty problem as from the clear evidence that the disease is on the increase worldwide. Researchers are tenacious and unswerving in their pursuit of an enigma, and this description of diabetes is extremely apt.

As medical science progresses in its unraveling of various mysteries, especially in the field of genetics, a new term has achieved considerable currency—genetic engineering. Scientists can now enter the womb of a pregnant woman through a process called amniocentesis, and by taking a sample of the amniotic fluid surrounding the fetus, can detect a number of genetic and congenital anomalies. By using this procedure and evaluating the findings, advice can be given the prospective parents about the possibility of bearing a defective child. In extreme cases, such as where the mother has had rubella (German measles) early in pregnancy, amniocentesis may be able to determine the extent of damage to the fetus. Thus the possibility of abortion could be considered if the impairment seems to be so extensive that the child might not be able to live a reasonably normal life.

Some progress has been made beyond this in the study of genetics, up to and including the identification of certain genes responsible for specific inherited conditions and characteristics. The ultimate aim of the geneticist is to be able to identify all of the genes and, perhaps through some biochemical means not yet discovered, modify those that may carry defects, anomalies, or diseases that are hereditary in nature. Diabetes, of course, is considered to be one of these. This is pretty far down the road, though, and smacks more than a little of *1984* and "Big Brother," Huxley's *Brave New World,* and even something of the legendary Dr. Frankenstein.

There is, however, a process carried on now to a certain extent. This is genetic counseling, in which an expert will perform tests and evaluate information to determine the possibility of parents' passing characteristics and conditions to their offspring, and will then advise the potential father and mother concerning the heredity pattern they may be creating.

Dr. David Rimoin said in 1973 that diabetes is the "geneticists' nightmare," so genetic counseling in this instance may not be as accurate as it is in other areas. He regarded textbook data on diabetic family histories as almost useless because they vary so much in terminology and in validity. He also said that medical science is dealing with a number of different kinds of diseases in diabetes in which environmental factors act on one or more genotypes (the fundamental constitution of an organism with all its hereditary peculiarities) to produce clinical diabetes. The counselor may therefore be at a loss to advise in a substantive way. That diabetes runs in families is an accepted theorem, but how it is transmitted is subject to a great deal of speculation.

Counseling one diabetic patient not to marry another and have children may eliminate their high-risk offspring, but if each marries a nondiabetic and they have children, the incidence of diabetes in the population will remain about the same.

"Only when we are able to define what kind of diabetes the patient has can we begin to make useful predictions," said Dr. Rimoin.

So—another attestation to the mystery surrounding diabetes. Not only is it baffling in its action but it offers the geneticists little satisfaction when they attempt to isolate an absolute mode of transmission from generation to generation, even though they are positive that heredity is a prime factor.

Research in genetics is progressing, however, at great speed, and scientists are now able to chart the human genes and chromosomes, which are the microscopic biological entities that provide the chemical basis for human identity. About 200,000 babies are born each year in the United States with some kind of birth defect. The annual toll due to these conditions is enormous, since several million Americans are affected by them and the hospitalization rate caused by genetically transmitted defects is high.

Study of the master chemical, deoxyribonucleic acid (DNA), that makes up the genes in which the messages of heredity are universally encoded has proved fruitful to the basic scientists. In 1961 the components of DNA were matched with their chemical functions within a cell. The genes are located in the 23 pairs of chromosomes containing the full set of instructions for body chemistry's role in making the individual human being.

At present more than 100 specific genetic disorders are known, each resulting from a single error in the chemistry of heredity. Since each of these leaves a trace in fetal cells, many can be detected long before a baby is mature enough for birth. The genetic component in other disorders that arise from a combination of factors is also better known, so that now at least 40 metabolic aberrations can also be detected early in the gestation period. It is possible to mark the chromosomes to show where the gene for a specific trait can be found. Within the next decade it may be possible to identify about 1,000 gene locations, and this should have a major impact on the knowledge of genetic diseases. With added knowledge concerning the causes of genetic defects, it may also be possible to alter genetic endowment deliberately and thus modify the inheritance pattern of the potential defect.

Should this ever be possible in application to diabetes, the means of preventing the onset of the disease could be at hand. True, the effect of all of this research may be decades away, but it cannot be denied as a wave of the future. Its accomplishment may imply modification of the accepted laws of heredity, but science is not above accepting new concepts even though it means discarding long-held ideas.

Should this bear a resemblance to science fiction, what of the future in tangible accomplishment regarding the treatment and management of diabetes mellitus?

From the public health standpoint, it should be readily apparent that more knowledge of the true extent of the disease is needed. This can be acquired only through comprehensive screening and detection programs undertaken on a nationwide basis, country by country throughout the world. Such projects should probe deeper into societal and life-style factors than by merely testing for diabetes symptoms. They should include nutrition habits, environmental influences, and viral causes as well as the determination of sugar levels in the blood and urine. Since it is well recognized that diabetes mellitus involves more than internal bodily mechanisms, an effort should be made in these surveys to delineate the influences of psychological stresses as well. Through these surveys the amount of occult diabetes would be determined, so that people who do not even know they have the disease can be brought into treatment.

The study of the disease entity itself is proceeding on two paths—basic and applied research. The first concerns itself with uncovering the prime cause or causes of the disease, and the second with methods of treatment and management.

It is in the area of basic research that progress is slow, painstaking, and as yet not very productive. True, basic research has provided some helpful information about various aberrations of insulin genesis and utilization. It has established that the two major types of the disease—juvenile-onset and maturity-onset—act in different ways. Medicine now knows that the juvenile's ability to secrete insulin is impaired almost completely, while the maturity-onset diabetic usually has some power to provide the hormone himself. It is also now known that other hormones, such as glucagon and somatostatin play an important role in the action of diabetes. Basic research has also revealed other manifestations that have significance in the development of the disease, and these are being investigated to determine their place in diabetes.

More and more emphasis is being placed on studying the receptor sites at which insulin does its work of enabling the cells to metabolize carbohydrate in a normal manner. The basic scientists are convinced that, where insulin is manufactured by the pancreas and yet diabetes does exist, the fault lies at one or more points in the process between the Beta cells and the receptor sites. Once this is determined, perhaps a means of correcting the aberration can be found.

Since it has been shown, statistically at least, that there is a relationship between mumps and a subsequent onset of diabetes, basic scientists are also investigating the possibility of viral causes of the disease. They would like to find out how a virus can affect the capacity of the Beta cells to produce insulin. If this becomes confirmed as a factor in the pathology of diabetes and exact effects of viruses can be elucidated, this might lead to a vaccine to prevent this kind of occurrence.

Additionally in basic research, the work is proceeding toward attempting to identify a marker for the disease that will indicate either its presence or future outbreak independent of symptoms of faults in the carbohydrate metabolism. The value of such a marker has been discussed previously, and a number of them have been alluded to, but so far none has stood the test of time. The more this is studied and the more that sophisticated methods are applied to this research, the better the chances of success if, in fact, a valid sign or signs exist.

Applied research appears to offer the most optimistic outlook for the short term in the treatment and management of diabetes. This is no doubt because this kind of research addresses itself to a specific problem, knowing what the defect is, and proceeds to devise a method for correcting it. The obvious failing in diabetes is usually a lack of insulin and the inability, no matter how insulin doses are juggled, to control the sugar balance. Thus the objective of applied research in this case is to provide the body with a continuing source of insulin that will mimic as closely as possible the activity of a normal pancreas.

Stimulated by the flush of enthusiasm for organ transplantation rife a few years ago, surgeons turned their attention toward replacement of the diabetic pancreas by transplantation. As was discussed earlier, this procedure was attempted a number of times but the results were disappointing in the main, because of the surgical problems inherent in transplanting the pancreas and basically because the rejection phenomenon common to all transplants could not be overcome. Some progress has been made since then in understanding the immunology of rejection, and it appears possible that at some future date pancreatic transplantation might become a more feasible method of treating diabetes than it is at present.

In recognition of the fact that it is the Beta cells in the pancreas that provide the insulin, some researchers have explored the potential of implanting these cells in the diabetic. The aim was to determine whether the healthy Beta cells would then vascularize themselves and continue to secrete insulin in their new environment. A number of experiments were performed in animals to find the best method for doing this, and it appeared that the portal vein of the liver was the optimum place for the implantation. There was some success for a time in diabetic rats, but eventually the Beta cells were rejected through the same reaction that caused rejection of the transplanted pancreases. However, where they were successful in the rats the implanted cells did provide insulin for a period equal to about one third of a rat's life. Should the rejection phenomenon ever be overcome, or should it be possible to prolong the life of the transplanted Beta cells for a significant time, this could become a treatment of choice in diabetes. And even if a group of these transplanted cells would survive for only a few years in a diabetic recipient before being rejected, it might be possible to perform the procedure again with new Beta cells, giving the diabetic another few years of his own internally manufactured insulin. This, too, is over the horizon of present knowledge. Immunologists are experimenting with methods of making the Beta cells more resistant to rejection through culturing them in various media before implanting them, and this, if some speculation is permitted, may prove effective in overcoming the problem.

Along with efforts at transplantation of the pancreas and the Beta cells, applied research is busy developing an implantable artificial pancreas, or Beta cell, if you will. This device, which would contain a glucose sensor, a computer for calculating insulin dose, a pump, and an insulin reservoir, is to be contained in a package smaller than a large egg. It is destined to be implanted beneath the skin, much as the cardiac pacemaker is now inserted, and through its action will provide insulin as the need is indicated by its instrumentation. The reservoir will contain enough insulin so that it would need to be refilled no more than once a week, or at longer intervals. Some problems surrounding this device, such as producing a cover for it that will not irritate surrounding tissue and ensuring that the insulin reservoir is absolutely leakproof, are being worked on now and are not considered impossible of solution.

There is little doubt that the end result of these efforts in applied research will be fruitful enough in the near future to offer the means of providing insulin in as physiologically sound a manner as possible, simulating the activity of the normal pancreas. When this is accomplished, the maintenance of the day-to-day, hour-to-hour balance of blood sugar should approximate that of the nondiabetic person. And what a boon that will be to the diabetic!

With good physiological control, with a diminution in the

wide variations in blood sugar levels observed even in diabetics supposedly in good control, the life of the diabetic should be considerably improved. There is mounting evidence, accompanied by wider acceptance, that good control of the blood sugar may well mitigate the occurrence of diabetic complications. Experiments in dogs that were made diabetic and kept under good control have shown that the sequelae so often seen in long-term diabetes did not occur, while those dogs in the control group who were barely kept alive manifested most of the microangiopathic changes, kidney failures, and eye involvements.

Thus, pending the discovery of the root cause of diabetes and the institution of measures to prevent the onset of the disease, the short-term outlook for diabetes appears bright. It must be emphasized, though, that until there is universal adoption of a method or procedure for ensuring good control automatically through one or the other of the means heretofore described, it is still up to the individual diabetic patient and his doctor to maintain the metabolic balance that will help to prevent, or at least modify, the dangerous and debilitating complications of the disease.

Whether this be by diet alone, by use of one of the oral hypoglycemic drugs, or through combinations of insulin, the diabetic will fare better under good control. He will live longer and will enjoy a more productive and satisfying life if he follows the kind of regime that his doctor and he have worked out to be in his best interest.

As society in general realizes fully the danger of diabetes, and as it menace is recognized by more and more people, the concern over its presence as a public health problem will grow apace. This will certainly be translated into demands for additional research, for additional consideration for diabetics, and for definitive answers to the as yet unfathomed questions.

Glossary

ACETONE—A substance formed in the metabolism of fat.

ACETONEMIA—The presence of acetone or acetone bodies in relatively large amounts in the blood.

ACETONURIA—The excretion in the urine of large amounts of acetone, an indication of incomplete oxidation of large amounts of fat.

ACIDOSIS—A high level of acidity in the body.

ALBUMIN—A simple protein widely distributed throughout the tissues of plants and animals. It may appear in the urine under certain conditions.

ANEURYSM—A circumscribed dilatation of an artery; a weak point in an arterial wall with consequent ballooning out of the vessel.

ANGIOGRAM—X-ray radiography of an artery after injection of a radiopaque material.

ANGIOPATHY—Any disease of the blood vessels; microangiopathy is disease of the very small arteries.

ARTERIOSCLEROSIS—Hardening of the arteries, a deteriorative process in which the walls of the arteries become thickened and lose their elasticity.

163

ATHEROGENESIS—The formation of fatty deposits in the arteries.

BASEMENT MEMBRANE—A continuous filamentous layer between the cellular lining and the underlying supporting material of body tissues.

CALORIE—The quantity of heat required to raise the temperature of 1 kilogram of water 1 degree Centigrade.

CATARACT—A loss of transparency of the lens of the eye.

CARBOHYDRATE—Chemical compounds that make up the most part of sugars and starches.

CEREBROVASCULAR ACCIDENT—Commonly called a "stroke" and resulting from damage to blood vessels in the brain, impairing bodily function.

CHOLESTEROL—A fatty substance found in the blood.

CESARIAN SECTION—Delivery of a baby by means of a surgical incision in the abdomen and uterus.

COMA—Loss of consciousness; in diabetes, resulting from very high blood sugars.

CORONARY—The name given to those arteries in the heart muscle which provide nourishment to that organ in its activity.

CYSTITIS—Infection of the urinary bladder.

DUODENUM—The first division of the small intestine arising out of the stomach.

DIURETIC—An agent that increases the amount of urine.

ELECTROCARDIOGRAM—A graphic record of the heart's action currents taken with an electrocardiograph.

ENDOCRINE—The internal secretion of a gland.

ENDOGENOUS—Originating in or produced within the organism or one of its parts.

ENZYME—A protein, secreted by the body cells, that induces chemical changes in other substances, itself remaining unchanged in the process.

ESTROGEN—A hormone, found normally in females, that produces growth of secondary sexual characteristics.

EXOGENOUS—Produced outside the body or organism.

GANGRENE—Degeneration and death of body tissue, usually caused by a lack of blood supply.

GASTROENTERITIS—Inflammation of the lining of both the stomach and intestine.

GLOMERULUS—The section within the kidney that filters waste products from the blood.

GLUCAGON—A hormone manufactured in the Alpha cells of the pancreas that acts to increase the amount of sugar in the body.

GLUCOSE—A form of sugar.

GLYCOSURIA—The presence of glucose (sugar) in the urine.

GLYCEMIA—The presence of glucose in the blood.

HORMONE—A chemical substance formed in one organ or part of the body and carried in the blood to another organ or part, which it stimulates to functional activity.

HYDRAMNIOS—The presence of an excessive amount of amniotic fluid in the womb during pregnancy.

HYPERGLYCEMIA—An amount of sugar in the blood that is above normal limits.

HYPOGLYCEMIA—An amount of sugar in the blood that is below normal limits.

HYPOTHYROID—Diminished production of thyroid hormone that results in certain clinical manifestations.

INTRAVENOUS—Within a vein or veins; when used in conjunction with "injection," it means that the substance is injected directly into a vein.

ISLETS OF LANGERHANS—Areas scattered throughout the pancreas that contain the Beta cells, which produce insulin.

KETONE BODIES—Substances formed during the metabolism of fat that are essentially acidic in nature.

KETOSIS—A condition in which acetone substances, or ketone bodies, are found in the body.

KETOACIDOSIS—Similar to ketosis, but found mainly in diabetics.

KILOGRAM—A metric system unit of weight equal to 2.2 pounds.

LIPIDS—A comprehensive term including those compounds which are insoluble in water and have the capacity of being metabolized in the body; the most common examples are fats and oils.

LIBIDO—Conscious or unconscious sexual desire.

METABOLISM—The process in the body that transforms foodstuffs into energy.

NEPHROPATHY—Any disease of the kidney, usually degenerative.

NEUROPATHY—Disorders of the nerves; when found in diabetics, such a disorder usually first manifests itself by a "pins and needles" sensation in the lower limbs, but it may take other forms.

OBESITY—An excessive amount of fat in the body.

OPHTHALMOSCOPE—An instrument used by the physician to examine the interior and back of the eye.

PANCREAS—The digestive gland located in the upper abdomen, behind the stomach, that produces both glucagon and insulin.

PHOTOCOAGULATION—The process of causing the coagulation of blood vessels by means of a light ray, specifically the laser beam, and used to correct blood vessel aberrations within the eye.

PITUITARY—A gland located deep in the brain that secretes a number of hormones that control other glands, as well as some body processes.

PODIATRIST—An expert in the care of the feet.

POLYDIPSIA—Extreme thirst.

POLYURIA—Frequent urination.

PREECLAMPSIA—An acute hypertensive disease peculiar to pregnant women characterized by high blood pressure, accumulation of fluid, and protein appearing in the urine.

PROTEIN—The basic structural substance of the body.

RENAL—Pertaining to the kidney.

RETINA—The inner layer of the back of the eyeball, which receives the light rays that enter the eye through the lens.

RETINOPATHY—Disease of the retina.

SIBLING—One of two or more children of the same parents.

STARCH—In reference to food, it is a substance that exists more or less throughout the vegetable kingdom, its chief commercial sources being the cereals and potatoes.

SUBCUTANEOUS—Under the skin.

SUBCLINICAL—Denoting a period in the evolution of a disease prior to the appearance of overt symptoms.

THYROID GLAND—An endocrine gland located in the neck that influences certain of the metabolic processes.

TOXEMIA—The clinical syndrome caused by toxic substances in the blood.

TRIGLYCERIDE—A combination of fatty acids found in the blood in certain circumstances.

UREMIA—An excess of urea and other nitrogenous waste in the blood due to failure of the kidneys.

VASCULAR—Pertaining to the blood vessel system in the body.

Index